The Managed Care Blues and How to Cure Them

The Managed Care Blues and How to Cure Them

WALTER A. ZELMAN
ROBERT A. BERENSON

Georgetown University Press
WASHINGTON, D.C.

Georgetown University Press, Washington, D.C.   20007
© 1998 by Georgetown University Press. All rights reserved.
Printed in the United States of America.
10   9   8   7   6   5   4   3   2   1   1998

Library of Congress Cataloging-in-Publication Data

Zelman, Walter A.
    The managed care blues—and how to cure them / Walter Zelman,
Robert A. Berenson.
            p.   cm.
    Includes bibliographical references and index.
    1. Managed care plans (Medical care)—United States.
2. Insurance, Health—United States.   I. Berenson, Robert A.
II. Title
RA413.5.U5Z44   1998
362.1′04258′0973—dc21
ISBN 0-87840-679-4 (cloth)
ISBN 0-87840-680-8 (pbk.)

                                                                98-16018

For our fathers

Benjamin M. Zelman
Whose nightly tales of politics and public life were charged
with a commitment to righting wrong and, just as importantly,
with an enthusiasm for the process.

and

Samuel J. Berenson
Whose unwavering professionalism remains an inspiration.

Contents

Preface   **xi**
Two Authors, Different Experiences x   Defending and Critiquing
Managed Care xiii

American Health Care:
Yesterday, Today and Tomorrow   1
The Long and Winding Road

The Old Non-System 6   The Logic of Managed Care 8
Managed Care under Attack 10   Fulfilling the Promise 12
Strategies for the Future 14

1
The Failure of the Old Insurance System   16
The Thrill is Gone

It Worked for All, except . . . 17   No Invisible Hand 18
The Tax Man Subsidizeth 20   Weak Buyers and Unique
Markets 21   The Costs of Scientific Advance 22   Self-Insurance
and the First-Hand Experience 23   Markets and Trade-offs 23
No Contest: The Government versus Costs 25   Controlling Costs,
Expanding Services 26   The Government versus Providers 27
Costly Compromises: The Birth of Medicare 28   Price Controls:
The Nixon Years 30   Providers Win a Pyrrhic Victory 31
Reinventing Medicare 32

2

Quality in the Old System: Not What We Thought   35

I've Been Loving You Too Long

Professionalism Will Do the Job 36   The Cottage Industry Cannot Adjust 37   Accountability 38   Practice Variation 39 The Information Explosion 42   Tolerance of Errors 43 Too Much Focus on Disease, Not Enough on Health 45 What Role for Professionalism? 46

3

The Rise of Managed Care   49

Birth of the Blues

Early Opposition 50   The 1970s and the Health Maintenance Organization 51   The Rise of HMOs and the Loss of Physician Domination 53   Managed Care Diversifies 55   New Niches and New Products 57   From Minority to Majority Status 60 The Trends Converge 61   The Clinton Plan: Managed Care and Markets Emerge Victorious 62

4

The Tools of Managed Care   64

You Can't Always Get What You Want

The Logic of Managed Care 65   A Taxonomy of Managed Care 66 Managed Care's Tool Box 68   Utilization Management and Preauthorization 73   The Tools in Action 82   Conclusion 86

5

The Cutting Edge of Quality Improvement   87

Good Vibrations

Quality Improvement Programs and Practice Guidelines 88 Demand Management 91   Programs for the Catastrophically and Chronically Ill 93   Disease Management 94   Specialty Benefit Carve-Outs 97   The Logic of Managed Care Meets Reality 98

6

The Managed Care Backlash   102
Stop in the Name of Love

Dissecting the Horror Story 105   Consumer Concerns: Who Comes First? 108   Choice, Access, and Quality 111   The Greed Factor 112   The Physician Backlash 115   Conclusion: Consumers at Risk 117

7

The Managed Care Record: Better Than You Think   119
Sympathy for the Devil

It Costs Less, and That Counts 120   Blame the System 121 Exaggerated Fears 123   Too Broad a Brush 126 Misunderstanding Value 128   Quality in Managed Care: What We Know and Don't Know 129   Consumer Satisfaction 134 Quality in Managed Care: They're Both Wrong 135

8

Rule of Price; Cult of Choice; Cost of Quality   137
You Better Shop Around

The Components of Value 137   Price: The Bottom Line Rules 139 Choice: of Physician, Plan, and Other Things 141   Quality: The Stepchild 151   Summary 158

9

Protecting the Floor   160
They Can't Take that Away from Me

Consumer Protection: Two Approaches 160 Approaches to Protecting the Floor: Some Wise, Some Not 162

10
Thirteen Steps to Raising Quality in Managed Care   179
With a Little Help from My Friends

1. From Employer to Employee Choice 179   2. Expanding
Consumer Choice to Delivery Systems, Not Just Insurers 182
3. Enhancing the Power of the Purchaser 183   4. Toward More
Cost-Conscious Consumers 186   5. Getting Sophisticated: The
Subtler Health Care Trade-Offs 188   6. Improving the Ability to
Choose: The Information Revolution, Part One 189   7. Improving
Clinical Performance: The Information Revolution, Part Two 193
8. From Opposition to Leadership: The Role of Physicians 193
9. Toward Greater Health Plan Liability: Another Approach to
Malpractice 195   10. Consolidation vs. Integration: An Antitrust
Challenge 196   11. Competing on Quality: The Devil in the
Details 197   12. A National Report on Health Care Quality 199
13. From Traditional Regulation to the Bully Pulpit 200

Epilogue   203
Bridge Over Troubled Water

References   205

Index   213

Preface

As liberals and Democrats we have often found ourselves in the uncomfortable position of defending two things many of our political friends distrust: managed care, and marketplace competition among managed care health plans.

Many would prefer that we focus on the abuses and failings of managed care and the need for government to impose more regulation on managed care plans and the marketplace in which they operate. They can't believe we would put much faith in competition among for-profit managed care organizations each of which can make more money by giving consumers less care and more impersonal service.

But if we followed the advice of our friends we would be telling only a piece of the managed care story, and probably not the most important one. Above all, our friends—and many others—tend to downplay the reality that managed care has significantly lowered health care costs. Lower costs have strengthened the nation's economy and freed up private and public money to address other needs—higher salaries, the lagging educational performance of our high school students, and health insurance for those Americans who cannot afford it, many of whom are children.

The reality, as we see it, is that managed care is not nearly as bad as our friends and others critics seem to think. Nor, we believe, was the system that managed care replaced anywhere near as good as many now want to remember. And, to the extent that managed care does need fixing—and it certainly does—it is far from clear that government regulation is the best or most potent tool for that task.

TWO AUTHORS, DIFFERENT EXPERIENCES

Both of us worked in the failed Clinton Administration health care reform effort. That's where we met. But aside from that common ground, our views about the potential of managed care derive from different perspectives and experiences.

Bob Berenson grew up admiring his father, a busy surgeon who was widely respected by professional peers and revered by patients. There was little question that the son would follow in the footsteps of the father. Trained as an internist, Dr. Berenson and a partner established a small, successful private medical practice in Washington, D.C., only seven blocks from the Capitol.

Starting his practice in 1981, Berenson was on the front lines when managed care swept over American medicine in the eighties. But, in contrast to most of his private practice colleagues, Berenson actually believed that managed care might be better than the traditional system. Why? First, the traditional system of paying physicians for every service rendered sent a number of wrong signals about practicing medicine. It produced a "blank check" mentality which encouraged, even rewarded physicians who ordered more tests or high cost procedures than may have been necessary; just as harmful, it penalized those physicians who spent more time with patients, diagnosing and understanding their medical problems.

In one memorable case, which began while he was on vacation, a physician partner referred one of Dr. Berenson's patients to a neurologist. The patient had complained of a slight numbness in some fingers on one hand. The neurologist recommended a battery of blood tests, various nerve conduction studies and three different MRI scans, a total of about $2,300 in tests. Properly suspicious, the patient decided to check with Dr. Berenson before going ahead with the tests. His condition, minor cervical spine arthritis, was then diagnosed with simple x-rays costing $50 and successfully treated with temporary use of a soft collar and aspirin.

Berenson's experience on various hospital quality assurance committees was also alarming. Many physicians seemed more concerned about protecting their autonomy to practice than with assuring the quality of care patients received. Specifically, these committees tended to explain away serious quality problems while strenuously arguing against any intrusion on the authority of individual physicians over medical decisions, regardless of their competency to handle certain cases.

On a more personal level, Berenson saw family members treated inappropriately by incompetent physicians accountable to no one for their mistakes and callousness. For his aunt had both diabetes and hypertension and had started passing out when standing up, risking serious injury. Her physician was prescribing an anti-hypertensive drug recommended to him by a pharmaceutical company salesman. Unfortunately, the physician didn't know what third-year medical students knew—that the drug was contraindicated (absolutely not be used) in diabetic patients precisely because it often caused large drops in blood pressure and fainting.

Finally, Berenson found the requirements of being a competent physician changing profoundly, and for reasons that had little to do with managed care. With the remarkable advances of medical science, the information physicians needed at their fingertips was growing exponentially. "Keeping up" by reading a weekly journal and attending an occasional conference was not longer sufficient. Moreover, patients were transforming themselves from passive recipients of physician efforts to active consumers, appropriately placing much greater demands on physicians' knowledge and communication skills. Instead of a narrow focus on identifying and treating disease, Berenson now found he needed to provide professional guidance to patients about preventing disease and managing the debilitating effects of chronic illnesses. These were new and complex professional challenges, tasks that raised serious questions about the viability of traditional medicine.

In short, Berenson liked managed care because it offered the chance to meet these new challenges and to transform the practice of medicine in a way that improved quality, increased physician satisfaction, and controlled costs. Of course, it has not always worked out that way.

Walter Zelman came to his views of managed care via a more political route. The son of politically active parents, Zelman grew up believing that all Americans deserved equal opportunity, a goal requiring government to lend many a substantial helping hand. Later in life, as a political scientist and California consumer advocate, Zelman spent considerable time and energy critiquing insurance companies on behalf of consumers and lobbying for reforms that would provide consumers more protection and clout in relationships with insurers. (In pursuit of that goal he even ran for the office of state insurance commissioner).

His interest in insurance issues eventually led to a position in the California Department of Insurance. There, among other things, he directed a task force of health care experts seeking a way by which California could guarantee health insurance to its over 6 million uninsured residents. He expected the task force (consisting largely of liberals and advocates of universal coverage) to advocate a Canadian-style, single payer system in which government would, among other things, set health care budgets and negotiate doctor and hospital fees. He himself had advanced such a position as a political candidate, and he held many doubts about managed care and market competition amongst managed care insurers.

But months of task force discussion and research led him to a series of rather different conclusions. First, it was clear that managed care was lowering health care costs, and lower costs would be critical if health insurance was going to be extended to many who could not afford it. Second, even if the American political system would tolerate a massive dose of health care cost regulation (and it probably would not), such regulation might not be the best long term means of controlling costs or protecting consumers. Third, managed care, properly conceived and implemented, had the potential to produce higher-quality health care than the status quo.

Thus, while Zelman remained attached to the goal of guaranteeing all Americans quality health care, he grew more open to market-oriented reforms comprising competition among managed care health plans to produce lower costs and better care. He began to think of such an arrangement as using the means (competition) associated with conservatives to achieve the ends (universal coverage) sought by liberals. That such an approach might actually offer up a viable political compromise was icing on the cake.

DEFENDING AND CRITIQUING MANAGED CARE

We suspect, we even fear, that what we have written here will be viewed by many as a defense of managed care. It is not. We, too, are critical of managed care, and disappointed in its performance to date. But our critique differs from the common complaints of consumers in the media. We are concerned that managed care is failing to improve the quality of American health care.

Not surprisingly, our view of the necessary solution is also different. We do not believe that the fix is a return to a pre-managed care system that both threatened to break the American bank and failed to deliver the quality of care consumers have a right to expect. Nor do we believe that the best fix lies in a long list of government imposed "do's and don'ts" that may ultimately limit both consumer choice and the ability of managed care health plans to improve quality and service. Rather, we believe a solution lies in finding the means (involving government, purchaser and consumer action) to make managed care companies live up to their potential for delivering higher quality, cost-effective care.

It is these different points of view and different assessments of managed care today that have prompted us to write this book. We believe many Americans may misunderstand managed care. We hope that policy makers, journalists, providers of care, and the concerned public will value a candid and balanced assessment of managed care today.

We offer just one caveat. We have not written this book for our colleagues in the field of health services research. We hope they will be interested in where we stand on some issues and in our analysis of some developments. But much of the material in the following pages will be familiar to them.

Nor did we seek to write a "how to" consumer book. Those looking for specific tips on "how to pick your HMO" or "how to protect your rights in an HMO" won't find it here. The audience we have aimed at is somewhere between those poles; those non-experts who want or need to know more about managed care—its origins, its record, its successes and failures, its potential, and what might be done to make it better.

A few words of gratitude are also in order. We want to thank Craig Havighurst, who provided us with high quality and invaluable assistance in structuring, restructuring and editing the text. His constant pressure to rethink and rework (while not always appreciated at the time) greatly improved the final product. We also wish to thank Jon Gabel, who shared a great many of his own insights into managed care and then reviewed the manuscript and offered a variety of comments and suggestions.

We also wish to thank the Washington D.C.-based Center for Health System Change, a project of the Robert Wood Johnson Foundation, for allowing us to use a number of charts originally printed in their publications and for producing an ongoing series of thoughtful discussions on marketplace change that have helped us test and develop our own ideas. Carolyn Martin and Moira Forbes provided valuable research and Internet search assistance. Our editor at Georgetown University Press, John Samples, offered time and the freedom to write the book as we saw fit. Our wives, Dr. Georgia Goldfarb, and Kathryn Berenson, provided considerable substantive and organizational input as well as the kind of critique that sometimes can only come from very special sources. To them we owe more than thanks.

Washington, D.C.
June 1998

American Health Care: Yesterday, Today and Tomorrow

The Long and Winding Road

Just ten years ago, most Americans knew almost nothing about managed care. They had never encountered a "gatekeeper." They knew little if anything about health maintenance organizations (HMOs) or preferred provider organizations (PPOs). Insured Americans went to the physicians and hospitals of their choice, and caregivers had few restraints on the kind or amount of care they delivered. Patients faced modest out-of-pocket costs and came to expect a steady stream of medical innovations and life-saving technologies as a matter of course.

It seemed to be a consumer-friendly system, but it had a fatal flaw. It could not control costs. In the second half of the 1980s, health insurance premium increases of 15 to 20 percent per year were commonplace. In 1990, it was considered *good* news when rates for employer-sponsored group health coverage increased *only* 14 percent; the year before, premium increases had averaged 24 percent (Sullivan and Rice, 1991). Health care spending consumed almost 13 percent of our national wealth (see figure on page 2). (Of twenty-nine industrial countries listed by the Organization for Economic Cooperation and Development, only the United States was in double digits on this measure [Anderson, 1997]). Soaring costs were undermining the competitiveness of American products in foreign markets and preventing workers from gaining meaningful wage increases. Labor negotiations no longer focused on how much wages might go up but on how much health benefits might have to go down. And the high cost of insurance was clearly contributing to the growing number of uninsured Americans, approaching 35 million by the end of the decade.

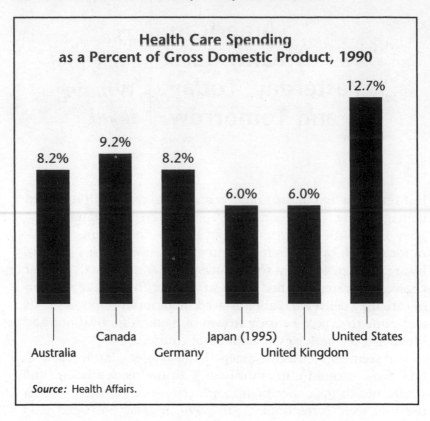

**Health Care Spending
as a Percent of Gross Domestic Product, 1990**

Source: Health Affairs.

By the beginning of the 1990s, it had become clear that, whatever the benefits it may have been producing, the American system of paying for and delivering health care was not sustainable. The repercussions of rising health care costs were simply too pervasive and too severe.

Today, just a few years later, that old system has undergone a minor revolution. Managed care has emerged from the shadows to become the dominant form of health insurance and delivery. By 1997, about 80 percent of Americans insured through employer-based insurance were in managed care plans. Growth in health care costs and insurance premiums has been under control—well below even the most optimistic of predictions. In fact, for three consecutive years in the mid-'90s, premium increases were actually lower than the inflation rate. In

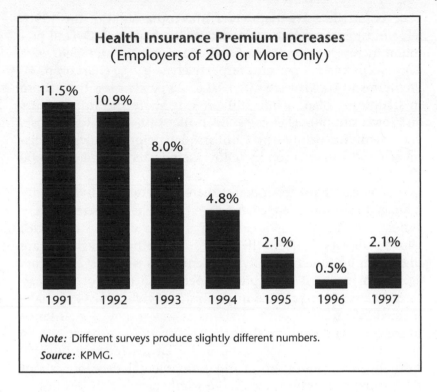

Health Insurance Premium Increases
(Employers of 200 or More Only)

11.5% 10.9% 8.0% 4.8% 2.1% 0.5% 2.1%

1991 1992 1993 1994 1995 1996 1997

Note: Different surveys produce slightly different numbers.
Source: KPMG.

the face of competition with managed care, the old fee-for-service system of health insurance is now withering away. In some communities it barely exists.

In difficult economic times politicians like to say that there are three issues in most campaigns: jobs, jobs, and jobs. Similarly, there were three issues behind the rise of managed care: costs, costs, and costs. Once managed care plans in certain parts of the United States began to demonstrate that they could lower those costs and, as a result, the premiums they charged, switching to managed care became almost a no-brainer, as they say, for employers and their benefits managers. They abandoned fee-for-service plans in droves, cajoling or forcing their employees to join HMOs and PPOs. The old system was, in fact, so inefficient and so antiquated that its collapse was very swift. When managed care finally came of age, it did so very, very quickly.

As for the costs themselves, the turnaround of the 1990s left almost everyone who watched it closely in awe. Overall premium increases in employer-based plans in 1995 and 1996 were 2.1 percent and 0.5 percent, respectively (e.g., see chart on p. 3). Premiums in HMOs were often 10 to 25 percent less than those in traditional plans while still offering more medical benefits and lower out-of-pocket costs. Even the scenarios of lower costs and premiums painted by Clinton plan reformers, widely dismissed as "fantasy" even by fellow Democrats, turned out to be conservative.

It is also hard to underestimate how deeply and broadly managed care has changed the face of the health care delivery system. Providers, the broad term used to describe hospitals, clinics, doctors, nurses, therapists, and other caregivers, are organizing in fundamentally different ways than just five years ago. In many areas, solo practitioners are a thing of the past. Most doctors now practice in groups. Individual hospitals have merged into multi-hospital systems of care, producing all kinds of concerns and hopes in the process. For-profit corporations, to the dismay of many, have extended their reach and influence. Insurance companies are facing fundamental decisions about the nature of their business. And a whole new line of business—managing physician practices—has emerged.

As one might expect, such sweeping change has not come without strife or controversy. While they may acknowledge the capacity of managed care to lower costs, many critics fear its impact on the quality of health care. They worry that health plans have too great an incentive to skimp on treatments for those patients who require the most care at the highest cost. They lament the loss of their cherished ability to freely seek care and choose their physicians at any time. State legislatures have considered and passed scores of proposals designed to keep managed care in check or to limit its impact. And the managed care "horror story" has become a staple of contemporary journalism.

In short, just about the time managed care became ascendant, it became a defendant as well.

This book, we hope, will put the debate over managed care into perspective—for the people who use it, who may one day use it, or who work within it. That debate has, we will argue, been driven and distorted by extreme points of view. Managed care's proponents tend to overstate its achievements: to date, they have made a better case about the merits of managed care in theory than in practice, and a better case for the ability of managed care to lower costs than for its ability to raise quality. Managed care critics, on the other hand, often provoked by media accounts that elevate horror stories over balanced analysis, have often forgotten or ignored the failings of the old system, while exaggerating both the threats and failings of the new one.

We will argue that managed care today is in fact neither snake oil *nor* cure-all. It is neither the danger that its critics charge it to be nor the panacea that its proponents claim it to be. It is better than the old system, but not nearly as good as it could be. We will explore how and why managed care has evolved, its multiple and changing forms, its current practice, how it is doing, its potential, and the means by which it might be improved. Our exploration will unfold in four parts that involve four main arguments:

First, the health insurance and delivery system we had before the advent of managed care was not nearly as good as many would like to remember.

Second, because it addresses many of the failings of the old system that preceded it, managed care has far more potential to control health care costs and to improve health care quality than the system it is replacing.

Third, while today's managed care plans have their short-comings, many of the most common criticisms one hears about them miss the point. The most serious failings of managed care today lie not in the restrictions it may impose on specific individuals at certain times, but in its failure to live up to its potential to improve the quality of health care for all.

Fourth, there are things that consumers, employers, providers of care, and government can do to increase the chances that managed care will actually achieve that higher potential.

THE OLD NON-SYSTEM

Nearly a century ago, George Bernard Shaw wrote in his preface to *The Doctor's Dilemma* "that any sane nation, having observed that you could provide for the supply of bread by giving bakers a pecuniary interest in baking for you, should go on to give a surgeon a pecuniary interest in cutting off your leg is enough to make one despair of political humanity."

Health researchers would begin to reveal in the 1970s that Shaw's droll commentary was not far-fetched. The old system gave providers the incentive to administer more health care than was really necessary. The more doctors did, the more they got paid. And many of them were clearly doing too much. Studies began to reveal that as many as 25 percent of invasive procedures were being performed without clinical justification. In other words, when judged against guidelines developed by experts and based on clinical evidence of what worked, those procedures were either "inappropriate" or "unnecessary" (Chassin and others, 1997; Kleinman and others, 1994; Greenspan and others, 1988). In another series of equally important studies, researchers found that many procedures were performed far more frequently in some communities than in others, but with no apparent effect on health status or medical outcomes. Apparently, many procedures were simply extraneous, adding cost and risk to patients while providing no medical value. What many did not realize, and still do not realize, was that the old system, consumer-friendly as it may have seemed, was failing on quality as well as on cost.

The critical point of such studies was not just that the practice of medicine was far from ideal, or that some doctors might be practicing it more wisely or judiciously than others. It was that *we didn't know*—that lessons learned about effective medicine were not always being passed on; that one community of medical professionals may not have known what another was doing.

These blind spots were one manifestation of another key failing of the old system: fragmentation. Most physicians practiced in independent offices, as individuals or as members of small group practices. There were few, if any, systems in place to monitor or evaluate provider performance, to communicate information among providers, to coordinate care in complex cases, to systematically assess what was and was not working, or to check the tendency for providers to do more than may have been appropriate or necessary.

In other words, the old system of fee-for-service insurance was no system at all. It may have laid health care on thick, but it often did so without finesse or efficiency. Consider a case study. One Sunday afternoon, author Berenson, then in private practice, got a call from the emergency room at the local hospital where he admitted patients. An eighty-two-year-old woman had fainted in church that morning and had been brought to the hospital by ambulance. She had experienced mild chest pain, and her emergency room electrocardiogram revealed that she had a heart arrhythmia called atrial flutter.

The patient was not able to explain much about her medical history, and there were no available medical records to help. She had not previously been in this particular hospital. Given her fainting spell, her chest pain, and the arrhythmia, Dr. Berenson saw no choice but to admit her to the coronary care unit (CCU) to make sure she had not suffered a heart attack. Tests showed she had not, and after an uneventful recovery, she was discharged after two days of hospitalization.

Over a period of six months, the elderly patient was admitted to four different hospitals with the same symptoms. In each case, the emergency department doctors—none of whom had any records on her previous admissions—admitted her to the CCU, fearing heart attack. To have done less might have arguably been substandard care. Overall, she spent twenty-five days in the hospital and had three full cardiac workups, including invasive testing to try to determine the cause of her abnormal heart rhythm. Each workup showed the same thing; she did not have a life-threatening cardiac condition, but rather a stable cardiac condition common for patients her age.

On her second emergency admission to the hospital where Berenson admitted patients—her fifth admission overall—the patient's granddaughter happened to accompany her. She explained that all of the spells had occurred on Sundays, in church. Piecing facts together, it became apparent that the patient would get very excited by the gospel singing that took place during the service and would then become faint. The mild chest discomfort and atrial flutter were chronic problems, completely unrelated to the spells and not life-threatening. The treatment called for had little to do with medicine or emergency rooms: she needed a chaperone to assure that she did not become overly excited in church. Instead, she received five admissions to hospitals and three expert—but expensive and totally unnecessary—cardiac workups, which were paid by her insurer, in this case the government-run Medicare program for the elderly, with no questions asked.

Consider the many inadequacies of this "non-system" of care. The patient did not have a regular physician who knew her, at least not one who could be identified and located. The various hospitals had no ready access to the patient's medical records. Each hospital and caregiver operated in isolation from the others; none had the information or history to recognize a pattern, let alone develop some kind of plan of care that would prevent any further unnecessary hospital admissions. And the payment mechanisms did nothing to discourage duplicative treatments. To the contrary, the providers actually profited from all the unnecessary care. The non-system generously rewarded highly trained physicians for performing expensive tests rather than competent clerical staff simply for locating family members or obtaining prior records.

In the end, this case cost Medicare tens of thousands of dollars, and the patient received vast amounts of unnecessary care when simple preventive measures might have solved the problem. To be sure, it was exploding costs, not poor quality of care, that undermined the old health care system. But as this case suggests, there were some serious and inherent flaws in that system. The way it delivered medicine is nothing to get nostalgic about.

THE LOGIC OF MANAGED CARE

The failings of American health care financing and delivery—its cost unconsciousness, its neglect of preventive care, its fragmented approach—were the fuel for managed care's rapid accel-eration in the late 1980s and early 1990s. Managed care proposed a new strategy and a new logic that would shake our health-care system to its core and rearrange the expectations of patients, doctors, nurses, hospital administrators, and every-body else associated with health care.

What did this new system offer that made its ascension so dramatic? At the most basic level it offered a remedy to unbear-able inflation. Without that, managed care would never have triumphed. But it had more to offer than just a capacity to reduce costs. It had the potential benefits of organization, coor-dination, integration, and the capacity, as a system, to learn and improve. Managed care would introduce new tools aimed at overcoming the failings of the old system and securing the goals of the new one. Patients would be directed into networks of physicians and hospitals whose practice patterns and outcomes could be reviewed; care would be better coordinated, usually by a primary care physician, who would act as a "gatekeeper" to more expensive and specialized services. The use of services by physicians and hospitals would be routinely reviewed, with the goal of increasing the probability that expensive procedures and hospitalizations would be performed only when necessary and appropriate.

And most important, new strategies of payment—in HMOs at least—would stand the old means of paying physicians and hospitals on their proverbial heads. Unlike the fee-for-service system, in which providers make more when they do more, pro-viders in HMOs may make more when they do less. This incen-tive, as we shall see, is a double-edged sword. Managed care's critics argue that the incentive to skimp on care is an unaccept-able answer to the profligacy of fee-for-service. We will explore that point of view in some depth, but for now we might want to think of prepaid health care as a powerful way to get health care organizations to think about keeping people healthy. Only under prepayment will health plans actually profit from educat-ing patients carefully about managing their own illness, encour-aging proper diet and exercise, keeping children on a rigorous schedule of vaccinations, or making invasive surgery the last resort that it often ought to be. This is not to say that doctors under the traditional fee-for-service system intentionally withhold information or immunizations. But neither do they have a record of going the extra mile in preventive care or of carefully weighing the health outcomes of low-cost techniques against more invasive and expensive ones.

Truly integrated care, in which the personal physician is one member of a larger health care team, has enormous potential both to reduce costs and to improve patients' health. The modern approach to treating asthma, for example, places devices and treatments in the home that a decade earlier were available only in the emergency room. With education and training, parents can act as surrogate nurses and physicians, performing medical tests, administering nebulizer treatment, and even adjusting medication—at lower cost, with less inconvenience, and with better outcomes for the child (Berwick, 1996). And now that it is becoming clear that the cause of asthma in many children living in inner cities is continuous exposure to cockroaches and dust mites, an asthma team dedicated to improving a child's health—or the health of a whole community—might even include an exterminator.

MANAGED CARE UNDER ATTACK

In spite of their successes, many leaders of managed care organizations must be scratching their heads today. They thought their success in reducing costs would have established their superiority over the non-system that came before. After all, policy analysts and, even more important, the employers who purchase health care are finally convinced that managed care saves money. Most have even accepted that, at minimum, its quality is no worse than the quality of the old system. Government is moving swiftly to put Medicaid (the government financed program for some very low-income individuals) recipients into managed care plans and, with a greater level of caution, to encourage Medicare recipients to choose the new system. In just nine years, the percentage of Americans with employer-sponsored insurance in managed care plans expanded from 25 to 80 percent.

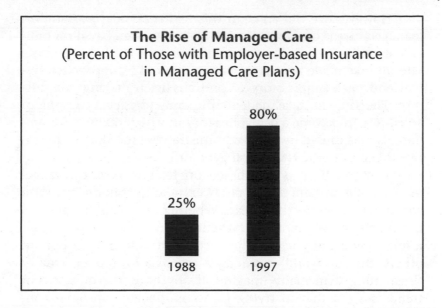

The Rise of Managed Care
(Percent of Those with Employer-based Insurance
in Managed Care Plans)

Yet, at the same time, managed care is facing an unprecedented assault—a backlash if you will—driven by charges and fears that the rush to lower costs will reduce patient access to needed care, choice of providers, basic consumer rights, and, ultimately, health care quality. In state legislatures and in Congress, literally hundreds of bills aimed at mitigating feared impacts of managed care have been introduced. Exposés of HMO "abuses," HMO hospital "muggings," or "consumers at risk" are appearing in all the media on a regular basis. Less restrained, New York City tabloids run stories reporting that, "Ex-New Yorker is Told: Get Castrated So We can $ave."

The fears of consumers are understandable and in some cases well founded. Certain approaches to paying physicians can lead to underservice that affects patient well-being. Significant restrictions on access to physicians of choice can threaten quality. Rules that attempt to restrict what physicians can tell patients about their medical needs are unquestionably inappropriate. Taken together, these policies and procedures can undermine the trust that patients need to have in their physicians and their healthcare-delivery institutions.

However, we will argue in this text that today's assault on managed care is often misdirected. It is too often based on individual stories or anecdotes that misrepresent the larger picture. The mistake made by a physician in the old fee-for-service system ends as a simple story of one physician making one mistake. The same mistake made by the same physician working in an HMO can become a page-one story in which the mistake supposedly was caused by some administrative procedure or incentive inherent to the HMO arrangement.

Today's attack is also based on fears of certain arrangements or circumstances that rarely exist, at least not in the form consumers or critics may fear. Whether the issue is financial incentives to save money, restrictions on choice of physician, limitations on physician-patient communication, or a host of others, the real world of managed care is a lot less extreme or threatening than many imagine. If anything, the most recent trends suggest that in trying to accommodate consumer concerns, managed care plans may wind up watering down their products to such a degree that the potential for real coordination and for cost and quality control may be lost. Today much of managed care—with expanding networks of physicians and groups, easier access to specialists, and in some situations, less intrusive utilization review—is beginning to look and act ominously like the old fee-for-service system, only with lower provider payment rates.

FULFILLING THE PROMISE

Managed care's track record on lowering costs is firmly established. But given the inefficiency and excess in the old system, cutting costs is not enough. What consumers want to know is whether individuals and populations are healthier under managed care than under the less restrictive fee-for-service system. Here the record of managed care is much spottier, especially when it comes to some of the most difficult cases such as the chronically ill and those with mental illness. In fact, the record reveals that when it comes to quality, managed care looks much better in theory than it does in practice. As a system, it has a long way to go before fulfilling its promise.

In the final part of this book, we will explore how we as a society can make our whole health care system better by making managed care better. This will be a collaborative effort involving health care providers, managed care companies, the government, employers, and, perhaps most importantly, the families and individuals on the receiving end of the health care system's many efforts. It will require finding a delicate balance between government regulation and market forces. It will require a reevaluation of the concept of choice: of what kinds of choices are really important and which may be less important. It will demand not just a strengthening of consumer protection rights in managed care—what we will call shoring up the floor—but the use of consumer purchasing power and savvy to force managed plans to improve the quality of care for all—or what we will call raising the ceiling.

The challenge of improving managed care will also require new practices and ways of thinking that get us beyond today's preoccupation with price. Health care purchasers have a lot to learn about assessing and comparing the quality of plans and about forcing managed care plans to compete on quality. More understanding is needed about the relationships between price, choice, and quality. And consumers must begin to ask themselves if choosing among plans might be more valuable than being forced into a single plan, even with its wide choice of physicians and other providers.

The stark reality is that in today's health care marketplace price rules. There are few market incentives for plans or provider groups to invest significantly in improving quality. And while plans have aggressively pursued market power through mergers and acquisitions, they have been slow to adopt the integration of care and caregivers that holds the real key to higher quality. To date, plans have been far more successful in applying the tools of managed care to lower price than to raise quality. As a result, managed care would appear to be falling far short of its potential to raise the quality of American health care, and it is here—not in the perceived reduction of choice or easy access to specialists—that the greatest shortcoming of the new system may lie.

STRATEGIES FOR THE FUTURE

Democracy, it has been said, is about the search for truth rather than about the truth itself. This is a useful concept with which to begin the effort to encourage, even compel, managed care to achieve its potential. It reminds all concerned that, whether we are discussing insurance and the organization of health care delivery systems, the markets in which they function, or government policies that set rules and frameworks, there may not be any definable set of ideal structures or solutions. In fact, a review of managed care organizations, regional health care markets, and government policies today suggests that all three are marked by enormous variation, experimentation, and ongoing change.

Under such circumstances, finding "silver bullet" solutions—for consumers, employers, providers, plans, or governments—will be difficult, if not impossible, especially if those solutions are geared to serve many circumstances over any length of time. For better or worse, solutions are more likely to come in the form of a relatively few broad sets of rules, goals, and strategies and a great many initiatives and ongoing adjustments undertaken by all kinds of actors.

We will endeavor to identify some of those rules, goals, and strategies, some of which may require government action. However, we will argue that neither government nor anyone else should attempt to define the ideal. Rather, we will suggest that government, purchasers, and consumers will be best served by policies and practices that encourage healthy competition and produce a variety of plans and health care delivery systems from which all can choose.

Each of these systems will entail a series of trade-offs between such values as cost, choice, quality, and even benefits. Some plans may offer trade-offs of less choice of physicians in exchange for a lower price. Others may offer higher levels of integration and presumably higher quality but with less opportunity to go outside the system. In the future, in well-functioning markets, some plans might even offer a heavy emphasis on prevention and treatments proven to be cost effective, combined with clear restrictions on very high-cost treatments that have a low probability of success. Other plans might offer easy access to such cutting-edge but costly therapies at a higher price.

Whatever the trade-offs allowed and offered, the critical factor is that the trade-offs be clear and that those making the choices have the necessary information to assist them in doing so. Only when trade-offs are clear will purchasers' decisions send the right messages to managed care organizations and others responsible for packaging and offering various trade-off decisions.

Gaining a better understanding of trade-offs is one of many things that consumers, employers, and government can do to become stronger and more savvy purchasers. If the marketplace, and not government, is to be the main agent of change, purchasers will have to know more and find the means to use that greater knowledge to increase their leverage in the marketplace. This may be especially true to the extent that they wish to push managed care plans to achieve their potential to raise quality. Here the questions may be not only *what* and *how* health care is purchased, but *who* purchases it. The "what" will involve better knowledge of the quality being offered; it may also involve the nature of the thing being chosen—specifically, whether it is an insurance company or a collection of physicians and/or hospitals constituting a delivery system. The "how" will involve the process of health care purchasing. The "who" will focus on the question of whether the employer or individual should be the purchaser or selector of plans.

In the end, to return to the original analogy of democracy as a set of choices, the recommendations we offer may read more like a constitution than a specific set of laws. American health care may be better served by managed care structures, competitive markets, and government policies that focus more on the ongoing search for truth—in this case, better health care value—than on the goal of concretely defining that truth.

1
The Failure of the Old Insurance System

The Thrill is Gone

The old system of health insurance and delivery broke down because it could not control costs. From 1965 to 1983, per capita health care expenditures grew 12.5 percent per year, nearly 5 percent greater than the underlying rate of inflation (Merrill, 1985). As early as 1967, President Johnson covened a conference on out-of-control health care costs. In 1971 President Nixon declared a health care cost "crisis," one that control did not abate until the mid-1990s. The inability of the system to slow down health expenditures undermined the nation's position in the international economy and kept wages from increasing. Even at this writing, with health care cost inflation seemingly under control, no one is certain that the genie will stay in the bottle.

The reasons behind the cost spiral in the old health care system are many, and they proved stubbornly entrenched in the face of decades of actual or proposed government action. In this chapter, we will explore the most important forces behind the cost explosion, including the insurance payment system in which a "third party" insurer pays the bill, the distortions produced by the favored tax treatment of health care benefits, the passivity and weakness of health care purchasers and consumers, the explosion of medical technologies, and the uniqueness of health care markets that left those who supply services in control of demand for them as well. We will then look at the government's tireless and virtually fruitless war on health care inflation. Understanding the shortcomings of the old system of health insurance, some of which persist even in the managed care era, should help us to understand why a new system emerged.

IT WORKED FOR ALL, EXCEPT . . .

Looking back, the flaws of the fee-for-service system seem so apparent that one is tempted to ask not why it collapsed, but how it survived so long. One answer is that to a large extent many participants in the system had no compelling reason to object to it: from where they sat, they liked what they saw. Most important, the biggest losers did not realize they were losing. Consumers, at least the ones who had insurance, had little to complain about. After all, they were largely free to go to any physician at any time and at little apparent cost to themselves. For the most part, employers paid insurance premiums and insurers paid the bills.

Physicians and other providers may have occasionally complained about insurers or governments that sometimes paid too little, but deep down they knew they had it made. Since no one shopped around for health services based on price, they did not have to compete with each other by lowering their fees. They maintained high incomes, succeeded in defeating virtually all government efforts to control costs, and maintained a stature and autonomy envied by virtually every other profession. They encountered minimal, if any, restraint in ordering tests or procedures for their patients because third-party insurance payment provided them with something akin to a blank check. This system even worked for insurers, for whom higher costs offered limited threat and real benefits. They passed on the higher costs to employers in the form of higher premiums and profited by having richer premium payments to invest.

Employers griped periodically about soaring costs but could do little about it. (Only toward the end of the eighties did they pass on the cost increase to employees.) Had these higher costs been obvious deductions from the paychecks of millions of Americans, the health-cost rebellion might have happened years earlier. But generally, the shifting of costs to employees came in the form of smaller wage increases over many years. Only as the relationship between stagnant wages and rising premiums grew more evident and more threatening to employer-employee relationships did employer concerns about rising contributions for health care coverage become a force to be reckoned with. When they did, the market began to get energized and the real rise of managed care began.

Even government, which pays close to half of the nation's health care bills, largely through the Medicare and Medicaid programs, found ways to limit its exposure to soaring health care costs. The Medicare program, in particular, set up systems in the 1980s to pay hospitals and then physicians less, fully aware that providers would make up the losses by charging others more.

Although they did not know it, the biggest losers in this blank-check, pass-through system were American consumers. They thought they were getting a lot for a little. But they were paying the bill in ways they never contemplated—in higher taxes, in higher prices on consumer goods, in lost wages, and in crowding out important investments in human capital and infrastructure. In this sense, they were the victims of a giant shell game that went on for at least twenty years.

NO INVISIBLE HAND

At the core of the old system stood third-party insurance, which can function like a recipe for inflation, leaving consumers virtually indifferent to the costs of care—especially when they most need services. In contrast to other kinds of purchases such as buying a car, consumers with broad third-party insurance coverage can go to the doctor with what feels like other people's—the insurer's—money.[1]

Moreover, while health care services usually entail some out-of-pocket costs for employees in the form of deductibles or co-insurance (e.g., 20 percent of the doctor's bill), most health care costs are paid up front, in the form of premiums. With virtually all of their costs already paid, consumers have little reason not to demand every test, procedure, scan, or other intervention, heedless of price.

---

1. Students of health policy will note that many employers self-insure, meaning that they bear their own risk. But to the employee, self-insurance is still insurance; someone else is paying the medical bills.

Students of economics quickly become familiar with the concept of the "invisible hand." Coined by English economist Adam Smith in the eighteenth century, the hand is the restraint the market imposes on any one provider of a service from jacking up prices or letting the quality of his service deteriorate. In a functioning market, that businessperson's clientele would simply go elsewhere. But in health care, insured consumers were not shopping with their own money, so they neither cared much about the costs being charged nor gave providers much incentive to compete by lowering prices. Nor did purchasers punish them for raising prices.

This lack of cost-consciousness on the part of employees was, and still is, rendered even more dramatic because families and individuals generally do not pay much of their own health insurance premiums. They are generally paid by employers as part of a total compensation package. In this way, health insurance is different from homeowner's, automobile, and most other kinds of insurance. In these forms of insurance, as with health insurance, the premium is paid up front, and there is no apparent reason for the consumer to demand anything less than the most they can receive for a claim—for an accident, a destroyed home, etc.

However, in other forms of insurance the consumer at least has the cost-consciousness that comes with paying the premium and thus more awareness of the relationship between premium costs, risks, and payouts. Indeed, many are so aware of the relationship that they decide not to report losses—such as minor automobile accidents—for fear that their premium will rise. And when it comes to public policy, they are more likely to sense the trade-off (in higher premiums) that may come with the passage of policy that offers more protection or benefits to consumers.

In markets without market discipline, complacency sets in and inefficiencies are allowed to fester and expand. Consider, for example, this story from the annals of President Clinton's health reform plan. In 1993, a director of a prominent academic medical center visited the White House and met with author Zelman, one of the individuals responsible for drafting the Clinton plan. "Before you decide to do too much," the director said, "you should recognize how much the marketplace is changing. Look, for example, at what our hospital has done in the last few years."

He then produced a series of charts revealing that in a relatively brief period of time his hospital had cut the number of high-cost procedures it performed and lowered its costs and charges by up to 40 percent. Charges at his hospital were now 15 to 25 percent lower than at the competing university hospitals in the same city. Careful review had demonstrated that neither the reduction in procedures nor costs had had any negative impact on outcomes or the health status of the patients.

One is tempted to ask: If a major medical center was able to reduce the use and cost of services so dramatically, without harming quality, what were they doing before making these changes? What kind of quality were they delivering? How did they survive, being so inefficient? Moreover, if its competitors were charging 15 to 25 percent more for the same procedures and performing them no better, how do those competitors survive? How long would a Ford dealer survive if he sold a Taurus for 20 percent more than a dealer a mile away? The answers were the forces of change described in this chapter. Purchasers and consumers of health care were not choosing based on price and quality, and physicians and hospitals were not being forced to compete on either. Costs did not have to be as low as they could be. It was a broken system.

THE TAX MAN SUBSIDIZETH

One may well ask why employers play such a large role in health care in the first place. The answer lies in war-time history. During World War II, employers used health benefits to attract scarce workers during a period in which wages were frozen. Immediately after the war, the rapid industrialization of America produced a booming economy that was able to generously provide new worker benefits, including health insurance. Then, in the late forties, the rapid growth of group insurance was fostered by a decision by the Internal Revenue Service that the employee's share of group health insurance contributions made by employers would be excluded from their income taxes.

The implications of this seemingly proconsumer and pro-health care public policy were profound. It made health benefits apparently cheaper than they actually were, and in so doing, it contributed mightily to the cost-unconsciousness problem.

The tax provision does not really matter to employers, who can deduct any compensation to employees as a cost of doing business. But for employees, the tax exclusion is a juicy plum. It acts essentially like a coupon good for a substantial discount off the costs of their health insurance. Offered another dollar in compensation by your employer, you could devote the whole dollar to better health insurance for yourself and your family or get a dollar minus state and federal taxes in cash (for most people about 65 cents) and then buy your own insurance. For most employees, the economics of the decision are fairly compelling: take the benefits. It seems like a good deal, but the tax exclusion makes it more difficult for employees to see the full cost of insurance. If they had seen that cost and the rates at which it was increasing, they might have been insistent that their employers do something about it and more understanding when they did.

WEAK BUYERS AND UNIQUE MARKETS

The tax wrinkle described in the previous section and the blank-check nature of health insurance conspired to make purchasers of health care, especially small firms and individuals, weak and unsophisticated. The nature of the insurance mechanism and of the product purchased (open-ended services, full choice of physician) seemed to leave all without the means or motivation to assert purchasing power. To consumers, all insurance products looked and acted pretty much the same. Most offered similar benefits, paid about 80 percent of medical bills (the consumer would pay the remainder), and allowed insured individuals to visit any provider. There was not that much for insurers to compete over, and there was not too much they could do to reduce their price.

And because insurers paid almost all of the bill, there was not much reason for consumers to pressure providers to lower charges. To be sure, insurers looked for ways to control the use of services and the prices paid for them. As costs continued to rise in the 1980s, insurers began to inform consumers that providers were charging more than the "usual and customary" fee, or that services provided were not "covered benefits" and that the consumer would have to pay part or all of the charges themselves.

But such actions hardly constituted the assertion of purchasing power by insurers. Insurers were not selecting providers for networks or negotiating fees. They would still pay any provider. At most, they would just force them to collect some of their fee from other patients. Moreover, since they could pass on higher costs in the form of higher premiums, their need to restrain rising costs remained modest.

Nor, it should be emphasized, did employers, employees, and insurers have much capacity to judge the value of what they were purchasing. Even today, there are few agreed-upon measures for the quality of health care provided by doctors, groups of doctors, hospitals, or health plans. Instead, consumers invested a good deal of trust and faith in the medical profession. We will see later why that trust may have been misplaced, but this phenomenon served to make the health care marketplace provider or supplier driven. Providers, in essence, both supplied the services and determined the demand for them.

THE COSTS OF SCIENTIFIC ADVANCE

At the same time that health insurance was expanding, medical science was making great strides in what it could do to combat disease and improve people's health. Today, in an era in which triple therapy with protease inhibitors offers promise of successfully treating even the HIV virus, it may be hard to remember that penicillin was not available until World War II. Compared to today, there was little that doctors and hospitals could do for people with serious diseases except try to make them comfortable while nature determined their fate.

However, after the war, medical science took off, discovering the means to treat and often cure diseases that had been deadly just a few years before. The perceptible reality of progress overwhelmed any theoretical concern about cost. To the extent that there was any political activity at all in health care, it was directed to trying to make medical care available to the many who could not afford it on their own.

Medical education reinforced the attitude among physicians that in their dedication to fighting illness cost did not count. The attitude was well encapsulated by economist Victor Fuchs, who, writing in the early 1970s, described physician behavior as following what he called the "technological imperative"—namely, the desire of the physician to do everything that he had been trained to do, regardless of the benefit-cost ratio (Fuchs, 1974). With the technological imperative firmly in place, and with the scientific capacity to do more soaring, general practitioners began to be replaced by specialists, who could more easily master the new technology and take advantage of the expanding scientific basis for medicine. But with specialization and technology came physicians' insensitivity to costs—they were busy saving lives.

SELF-INSURANCE AND THE FIRST-HAND EXPERIENCE

Under such an inherently inflationary system, it should come as no surprise that those who were first to rebel were employers who self-insured, that is, who paid medical bills directly rather than purchase insurance. They might have passed some costs on to employees, but they saw both the origins and results of soaring costs first-hand. They also saw how dramatically they—and their employees—might benefit if those costs could be reduced. In the 1980s, some would become both aggressive and creative in trying to get those costs under control. But even the largest of them would not have the success that managed care organizations would soon experience.

MARKETS AND TRADE-OFFS

A common theme runs through all of these causes of runaway costs: health care has not been bought and sold like other goods. Typically, supply and demand push and pull one another over time until prices settle at an equilibrium point that reflects society's willingness to pay for something and producers' willingness to provide it. But until very recently, in the health care marketplace, providers (suppliers) wielded most of the power. They determined need (demand) for and quantity of services to be supplied and then set the price. People did not "demand" or desire CAT scans or brain surgery, and they did not ask the price. So the forces that would ordinarily check spiraling costs were either absent or weak.

Moreover, in other markets consumers often settle for what they need, rather than for what they may want. They accept trade-offs between cost and other factors. They may want a larger home, but their financial resources or other needs compel them to accept a smaller one. They may want to purchase an expensive designer suit but decide that the one from Sears will be adequate. Health care markets were, and to some extent still are, different. Insured patients have not had to confront similar trade-offs in choosing among health care providers or modes of care.

This is changing today. Managed care is confronting Americans with difficult trade-offs that many have been able to avoid or ignore for years—for example, the trade-off of lower charges in premiums and medical bills in exchange for less choice of provider. But many consumers still do not see themselves as carrying the full burden of health care costs. Consequently, they are less concerned than normally would be the case about things that might drive up those costs and less likely to accept the trade-offs involved in lowering those costs. The additional costs, for example, of a forty-eight-hour as opposed to a twenty-four-hour hospital stay after giving birth, of increased home health care benefits, of easier access to specialists, or of insurance coverage of unproved, experimental procedures are still seen as being paid largely by employers or insurers.

Similarly, consumers may be less likely to see the value in lower health care costs achieved in managed care arrangements. Those lower costs will be viewed as benefiting employers, who will pay lower premiums, and insurers, who may make more profit.

For the promoters of managed care plans, these realities leave them behind the proverbial eight ball. Their greatest proven asset—the ability to lower costs—is grossly undervalued by consumers, who remain much more alarmed about the restrictions managed care may impose than they are pleased with the lower costs it has produced.

NO CONTEST: THE GOVERNMENT VERSUS COSTS

Early in his first term in office, President Richard Nixon told a news conference that rising health care costs in the United States constituted a "massive crisis." "Unless action is taken within the next two or three years," he asserted, "we will have a breakdown in our medical system" (Starr, 1982). It was not the first time a U.S. president had fretted openly about the state of health care costs. But it did mark the beginning of a new era in which words like "crisis" and "breakdown" became standard rhetoric in discussion about the American health care system.

Nixon was referring to both public- and private-sector costs. Businesses were frustrated as they watched the price of insuring their workers rise inexorably. The Medicare and Medicaid programs, then just a few years old, had already started to look like fiscal black holes, absorbing ever larger portions of government budgets. The forces of supply and demand that keep prices in check in the rest of the economy just would not or could not restrain the blank-check, fee-for-service health care system.

Under such circumstances we might expect that in America it would be the marketplace, not government intervention or regulation, that would be the first line of defense against rising prices. But, as outlined above, health care did not fit most market scenarios. The blank-check, fee-for-service system offered few means by which markets could control costs. The pass-through insurance system shielded consumers from the real costs (in wages) of health inflation. Employers who might have otherwise rebelled were able to pass much if not all the increases on to employees. Moreover, there was widespread doubt about the wisdom of promoting competition amongst health care providers; market pressures, it was feared, might undermine their commitment to a patient-first ethic. Only a few far-sighted individuals presented a vision of market-oriented approaches to health system reform and cost control. Indeed, the most influential of market-reform theories, dubbed "managed competition," did not appear in print until 1978, (Enthoven, 1978).

As a result, leadership on reducing health care costs was left largely to government, at least until well into the 1980s. Many government leaders would try to get the job done. Just about all of them would fail.

CONTROLLING COSTS, EXPANDING SERVICES

Government, it turns out, was responsible for much of the health-cost problem. In 1965, Lyndon Johnson and Congress provided universal health insurance coverage for the elderly through Medicare and coverage to many of the poor through Medicaid. These programs helped fill glaring needs in American health care, but controlling their costs posed Herculean tasks. In Medicaid, the need to control costs conflicted with the desire to expand coverage to more poor people and a booming demand for nursing home coverage. In Medicare, the problem would lie in the adoption of the fee-for-service system and in the vigorous opposition of a politically powerful senior citizen community to any changes that might either increase what they had to pay or decrease the benefits they might receive.

Other government efforts would exacerbate the health care cost-control problem. Washington funded tens of billions of dollars' worth of health research, which spurred the biotechnology industry to achieve remarkable breakthroughs against deadly and disabling diseases. But the ability to do more, however valuable, would come with a high price tag in health care spending. The federal government responded to pleas from millions of Americans in rural and inner city areas without family doctors, subsidizing medical education to produce more doctors in the hopes that some of them would locate in underserved areas. Some did, but many more settled in affluent areas where they were not necessarily needed and where they generated lots of additional spending on health care because of the fee-for-service system. Physician oversupply was eventually deemed so serious that after decades of contributing to an excessive physician workforce—most particularly an excess of specialists—Congress enacted legislation in 1997 that essentially pays medical schools *not* to train physicians, much like the federal government has paid farmers not to produce crops.

Government would also subsidize hospital construction and continue to do so even after it had become clear that the nation had too many hospitals. And it would, as discussed earlier, continue to put employee health care benefits on sale relative to other goods and services by excluding them from taxable income.

The pros and cons of these and other actions could be debated. What is not debatable is that the net effect of these and other actions was higher and higher health care spending.

THE GOVERNMENT VERSUS PROVIDERS

When government did try to control costs, its efforts would almost always encounter political hostility. Federal efforts were attacked as interference with professional autonomy, as inappropriate manipulation of the market, and even as "socialism."

The record that emerged stands in marked contrast to the experience of health care cost control in other industrial democracies. Policy makers in those countries have gone much further than those in the United States, both in guaranteeing access to care for all citizens and in placing direct controls on the flow of money through their health care systems. By limiting the expansiveness of the health care infrastructure, for example, the number of hospital beds and expensive technology such as MRI facilities; by assuring that most medical students practice as generalist physicians, not as specialists; and, in some cases, by negotiating or dictating payment rates for physicians and hospital budgets, other countries have spent much less than the United States on health care, whether measured as a percentage of gross domestic spending or as per capita costs.

Projected Surplus of Specialists in Year 2000
(By Percentage of Excess)

Neurosurgery	57–196%
Plastic Surgery	125–177%
Cardiology	53–114%
Anesthesiology	74–95%
Ophthalmology	57–90%
Neurology	53–82%
Radiology	42–68%
General Surgery	52–63%
Gastroenterology	48–55%
Orthopedics	20–52%

Source: JP. Weiner, *JAMA*, July 20, 1994.

American providers, however, drawing on their political strengths that resulted in part from their contributions to the political parties; their credibility as professionals; the innate hope of consumers that their physicians knew best; and long-standing American fears of government intervention and regulation fought government cost-control efforts at every turn, and with remarkable success. Whatever the merits of their arguments, their success only exacerbated the cost problem.

COSTLY COMPROMISES: THE BIRTH OF MEDICARE

The passage of Medicare and Medicaid in 1965 were giant steps in American history. Both programs represented new and laudable commitments to needy populations. But both were constructed and further fortified on the foundation of the old fee-for-service system. The next twenty years would be marked by tension between the need to maintain and even expand these programs and concerns about the costs they generated.

In the case of Medicare especially, the blend of new program and old payment system would prove particularly volatile. Whereas states, which administered the Medicaid program, were prepared to impose dramatic controls on fees paid to physicians treating the poor, it would be almost a decade before any such controls (and even then only modest ones) were imposed in the Medicare program. In Medicaid, costs rose rapidly because more individuals were made eligible for the program and because the numbers depending on Medicaid to pay for nursing home care soared as well. In Medicare, costs grew largely because spending per individual spiraled upward.

Medicare's inflationary ways were the product of its original design, which in turn was a product of politics. Despite the manifest need for the program to provide structured health insurance coverage for seniors, the American Medical Association (AMA) had pulled out all the stops to oppose its passage, calling up the shopworn but still effective specter of socialized medicine. To overcome that opposition, political leaders had to ignore or abandon any concerns about cost control or accountability of physicians. President Johnson directed aides to give the AMA what they wanted. Among other things, what the AMA wanted was language in the 1965 Medicare statute that prohibited the federal government from exercising "any supervision or control over the practice of medicine" and that adopted a highly inflationary payment system that essentially paid physicians based on their own charges and not on a reasonable and controllable fee schedule. To guarantee quick national acceptance of the program, the Johnson Administration established policies and procedures for hospital and physician payment that were generous to the providers. In short, to achieve political passage and initial acceptance by a critical medical profession, Medicare was enacted without effective mechanisms for restraining costs.

Medicare provided an explosive mixture of pent-up demand for services, providers ready and willing to satisfy that demand, and the absence of virtually any provisions to restrain cost increases. The fiscal result was inevitable. Medical cost inflation rose from a little over 3 percent before Medicare to 7.9 percent annually in the five years after Medicare's enactment. In later years, it would get even worse. When the costs of Medicaid were added in, the impact on government budgets was even more dramatic. Between 1965 and 1970, government's share of national health expenditures jumped from 26 to 37 percent, reflecting an annual rate of increase in state and federal expenditures of nearly 21 percent (Starr, 1982). By 1995, government's share of national health spending would be 45 percent, with the federal government's share comprising more than one-third of the total (Health Care Financing Review, 1996).

PRICE CONTROLS: THE NIXON YEARS

Nixon was the first of many presidents to try to achieve some control over health care costs, initially as part of his imposition of a general wage-price freeze on the economy in 1971. By December 1971, the wage-price program strictly limited rates of increase in doctors' fees and hospital charges. Even when general price controls were lifted from most commercial sectors in January 1973, those imposed on health care were retained. The freeze was temporarily successful in holding down health care costs, but when the controls were finally lifted in April 1974, health care inflation rebounded.

The failure of Nixon's price controls did not stop others from undertaking efforts to police health care spending. Most notable among these were programs launched in the early 1970s that become known broadly, and later pejoratively, as "health planning." In order to exert a kind of proxy control over health care spending, a number of states established programs to control the capital expenditures of hospitals and nursing homes by requiring these institutions to obtain state approval called "certificates of need" for construction projects and other large capital investments. In essence, these programs asked quasi-public planning agencies to pick winners and losers among competing claims for capital improvements. But facing inevitable political opposition from potential losers and succumbing to politically inspired loopholes, most health planning programs were either scrapped or scaled back to virtually nothing by the 1980s. Subsequent research indicated that they had been largely ineffective (Salkever and Bice, 1979, Sloan, 1988).

Other approaches to cost control included state programs to directly regulate hospital rates or to establish physician-review organizations to modify the care provided by their physician peers. A few achieved some success. Even fewer, such as Maryland's hospital rate-setting efforts, had considerable success. But most would either fail or become unsustainable because of political opposition.

PROVIDERS WIN A PYRRHIC VICTORY

Like Nixon, President Carter would pick up the mantle of health care cost control. And like Nixon, he was not able to carry it very far. Upon assuming office in 1977, the Carter Administration immediately identified hospital cost containment as one of its most important domestic policy initiatives. Under this proposal, the federal government would attempt to restrain costs not only in government-run health care programs, but in private-sector insurance programs as well. Although primarily focused on the need to reduce bulging budgets in government entitlement programs, including Medicare and Medicaid, the administration was concerned that the application of spending limits to only Medicare and Medicaid patients would result in cost shifting to purchasers of health care in the private sector. That is, hospitals could attempt to recoup from private payers what they no longer were permitted to collect from government purchasers. As a result, supporters asserted, unless cost controls were placed on both public and private spending, the overall rate of health care costs would rise unabated, to the detriment of the economy and the competitive position of American industry.

Carter's proposal to Congress would have imposed hospital budgets from the top. It would not have attempted to micromanage the decisions of doctors or control clinical decision making. Even so, providers and others attacked it as bureau-cratic, government-run medical care. Although Harry and Lou-ise—the fictional couple that would later emerge in TV advertising as effective critics of President Clinton's health plan—would have been only teenagers at the time, the criti-cisms of President Carter's Hospital Cost Containment legisla-tion were similar to those that helped defeat Clinton's Health Security Act almost twenty years later.

To provide their congressional supporters with political cover while they killed the Carter proposal, the American Hospi-tal Association, the AMA, and other provider groups undertook a "Voluntary Effort" effort to hold down hospital costs. But to the surprise of few, the effort proved feeble and ineffective. Hos-pital Cost-Containment legislation was defeated in Congress in 1979, and when the election of Ronald Reagan in 1980 finally eliminated the threat of similar legislation, hospital costs resumed their upward trend, but at unprecedented rates. From 1980 to 1983, in the immediate aftermath of Hospital Cost Con-tainment's defeat, health care expenditures increased by nearly 14 percent per year, which, even during a period of high infla-tion in the general economy, represented a 5 percent real rate of growth (Merrill, 1985).

Whether the Voluntary Effort had been a political ploy or a serious provider initiative, its failure had important repercus-sions. It would demonstrate to purchasers that voluntary attempts by organized medicine and the hospital industry to impose cost discipline on its members were not the answer to soaring costs and, in all likelihood, never would be.

REINVENTING MEDICARE

By the 1980s, general health care costs were a major concern, but Medicare's costs represented a nightmare unparalleled. Costs had exceeded the program's original estimates by five or six times, and providers were racking up exorbitant profit margins on the backs of taxpayers. In the early 1970s, Congress had altered payment rules to place some limits on what it would pay physicians, but the limits imposed were quite modest. The problem was easy to diagnose but hard to fix politically.

"Only Nixon could go to China," says one bit of standard political wisdom. Perhaps, then, it should not be so surprising that it was under the Reagan Administration that, amidst all the rhetoric of getting government off the backs of the American people, government took its first really significant steps to rein in health care costs. In 1983, the Reagan Administration struck a deal with Congress to fundamentally change the way Medicare reimbursed hospitals. Instead of reimbursing the costs that hospitals had incurred in caring for a patient on a fee-for-service basis, a new Prospective Payment System would now pay a fixed fee for each hospital admission, based on the patient's diagnosis. Whether the patient stayed two days or ten days in the hospital, the Medicare payment to the hospital would be the same.

The new program, which had much in common with prepayment concepts emerging in HMO plans, set in motion an important series of changes and sent new signals to all the major players in health care. For the Medicare program, the switch to fixed, predetermined fees for hospital stays meant that for the first time Medicare could gain a measure of control over the budget for hospital care, which at the time comprised more than two-thirds of Medicare spending (Crozier, 1984).

For hospitals, the new reimbursement approach completely altered financial incentives, at least for Medicare patients. Under the old payment system, doing more—longer stays, more procedures, etc.—produced more revenues and presumably more profit. Under the new system, doing more would generate only higher costs, not higher revenues, and reduced profits. In short, given the same patient with the same diagnosis, doing less and at lower cost was now better.

Finally, for private-sector purchasers, the new Medicare payment mechanism sent a strong, albeit perhaps more subtle, signal. In distinct contrast to President Carter's Hospital Cost-Containment legislation, which would have imposed regulatory controls on both public and private hospital costs, the new Medicare payment rules would apply only to Medicare purchasing. The government, in other words, was going to take care of only its own problem. As the new rules took hold, private-sector employers began to understand about cost-shifting from Medicare to private-sector insurance. From the employer's perspective, then, a bad situation was only getting worse.

As double-digit premium increases continued, the only other thing employers could discern just on the horizon, was the potential of emerging managed care organizations to provide a cost-containment option. Fortunately for employers, those organizations were beginning to demonstrate the potential, if nothing else, to control costs. Thus, as the old system was cracking, a new one was beginning to demonstrate its worth.

2

Quality in the Old System: Not What We Thought

I've Been Loving You Too Long

We hope we have established that under the traditional insurance system, health care costs were soaring upwards at unacceptable, even unconscionable, rates. The fee-for-service system provided a blank check to insured patients and providers, who unwittingly conspired—with what may have seemed to be justifiable motives—to spend the nation into a cost crisis.

Throughout this period, however, American health care maintained a reputation for being of the very highest quality. We may have paid the most—some 25 percent more per person than any other nation—but at least we got the best, or so we assumed. In some respects, we were probably right. For example, in the development and application of high-tech medicine, American medicine had no peer. Yet, by many measures, such as infant mortality rates and life expectancy, the performance of American health care was somewhere in the middle compared to other modern industrialized countries. Actually, for all of the assumptions about American health care superiority, we really did not know much about the quality of care we received. We had no established set of national guideposts with which to rate the system's performance or to compare doctors or hospitals. Instead, we deferred to the medical profession to run the system; we assumed they were performing well because that's what they told us. Eventually, researchers would begin to find some answers to the how-good-is-our-health-care question. The answers were not very reassuring.

PROFESSIONALISM WILL DO THE JOB

The assumption of high quality in American medicine may have rested on a pillar of faith. We believed that medical knowledge and competence rested on a body of rational and scientific information, that physicians were dedicated to maintaining their technical knowledge and competence, and that doctors would establish rigorous peer review procedures to keep each other on their toes. In short, we believed that *professionalism* ensured quality. Physicians would act in the best interests of patients, we assumed, because their professional ethic required them to.

Until relatively recently, these admirable professional attributes seemed to serve the public well. The Marcus Welby-style physician had real-life counterparts who through hard work and dedicated patient service solved their patients' medical problems, or at least held their hands when nothing could be done. But Marcus Welby practiced in simpler times—before the blizzard of scientific breakthroughs that provide seemingly miraculous cures but that now require physicians to be absolutely up-to-date; before the era of consumerism in which patients no longer are willing to accept paternalistic assurances of physicians that they know best; and before the country arrived at a collective decision that it could no longer give physicians and other health professionals a blank check to do what they thought best (which, by the way, also served to maximize their own incomes).

Perhaps this last factor—the medical profession's lack of interest in holding down costs, whatever the high-minded philosophical rationale or ethics underlying it—was the decisive one that would eventually undermine the old system and the profession that benefited from it. With the change would come a substantial challenge to the dominance and autonomy of the medical profession. That challenge would extend well beyond the organization and regulation of the profession to the physician's control, once viewed as nearly total, over clinical decision making for individual patients.

Looking back, it is clear that the medical profession never lived up to the ideal of the model. As one analyst recently concluded, "The myth of a lost 'Golden Age' of medicine before the advent of managed care should be rejected. Marcus Welby isn't just dead; he never lived . . ." (Millenson, 1997b). In particular, it has become clear that as a means of assuring all high-quality care, professionalism—based as it was on the presumed integrity, commitment, and skill of the individual practitioner—even if once plausible, is no longer adequate. Medicine has changed too much. Even Marcus Welby would find the task too imposing.

THE COTTAGE INDUSTRY CANNOT ADJUST

Until very recently, medicine in the United States was organized as a cottage industry. Solo doctors practiced as small-businessmen. (Until the last two decades, there were relatively few women physicians.) A doctor hired his own staff, determined his own work schedule, set his own fees, maintained records for his own use, and had informal, collegial relationships with other physicians. Patients were free to shop around for a physician they admired, with few restraints on their choice. They did this, however, without objective data to help them make their decisions. And because of ethical strictures imposed by professional organizations including the AMA, physicians did not advertise their own services.

Thus, picking a doctor was, and still is, based largely on word of mouth. Recommendations usually came from family members, neighbors, or fellow workers, and more recently from disease-oriented support groups and even "best doctors" surveys published in local magazines. Specialist referrals were recommended generally by the treating doctors themselves. If patients did not like the care they received, in the fee-for-service system they were free to move on to another physician, with no one else the wiser.

In some ways, this improvisational approach to pairing up doctors and patients worked reasonably well. In conventional, open-choice insurance, patients enjoyed the prerogative to exercise their own judgments about physicians and therefore tended to be happy with the physicians they settled on. Indeed, public surveys demonstrate that individuals are still satisfied with the care *they* receive but consider the performance of the health care system overall to be wanting. Put another way, patients have a natural tendency to trust their personal physicians, even if they are critical of the medical profession as a group.

But there was a price for this freedom. For much of its history, medicine was viewed as more art than science. There was little objective data with which to measure the quality of care doctors provided. Patients tended to respond more to doctors' personalities and attentiveness than to any measurable level of their proficiency. Patients' need to trust their personal physicians was so great that even when things went badly, patients often would not go elsewhere. As a result, patients may have invested too much trust in the idea of the autonomous physician.

To be sure, doctors rarely act out of base motives or display incompetence. The point is that health care has simply become too complex to assume that a well-meaning physician, acting alone, is capable of providing the high-quality care patients need. The evidence comes in many forms: reliance on professionalism alone may not be enough to guarantee that care is of the quality that patients and society need.

ACCOUNTABILITY

In the cottage industry that preceded managed care, a doctor faced little or no formal accountability to external parties for the quality, cost, or any other aspect of the medical care he or she provided. If something went extremely wrong, of course, he may have been sued for medical malpractice for allegedly violating accepted professional standards of care. In even rarer circumstances, patterns of incompetence may have resulted in limitations on his license to practice medicine or on his hospital privileges.

The lack of routine accountability began to change with legal doctrine established in the 1960s that held hospitals corporately liable for many of the in-hospital activities of physicians to whom the hospitals granted privileges. In response, hospital medical staffs developed improved peer review programs that provided a degree of scrutiny over physician performance for hospitalized patients. Medical care provided in offices and clinics outside of the hospital, however, was rarely subjected to any review at all. State licensing authorities, established to assure the public that licensed professionals possess a basic level of competence, were usually dominated by physicians who did not take well to sanctioning their colleagues. Accordingly, the licensing authorities compiled poor records of intervening to restrict practice or even to conduct remedial, educational programs. They represented, in many cases, classic examples of well-intentioned regulations being coopted by the regulated and thereby rendered ineffective.

Another presumed source of accountability was the malpractice system, which was supposed to act as an external deterrent to poor practice. Yet few knowledgeable observers today believe that the malpractice system does much to weed out incompetent physicians or raise overall levels of care. Research has found that very few negligently injured patients actually bring a malpractice suit. In the largest study of its kind, only 3 percent of hospitalized patients who appeared to have suffered a serious negligent injury actually brought suit (Localio and others, 1991; Burstin, Lipsitz and Brennan, 1992).

In short, in the cottage industry that managed care is replacing, a medical license was essentially a guarantee of a lifelong opportunity to practice with little oversight or accountability. Because much health care has migrated out of hospitals, where at least basic peer review does take place, the public now would have even less assurance that physicians actually were practicing within their levels of competence. It all depends on the integrity and commitment of individual physicians, and that has proven highly variable.

PRACTICE VARIATION

It is hard to imagine that in a society that measures, quantifies, and standardizes just about everything, medicine, is rooted as much in folkways and tradition as in hard science. In the late

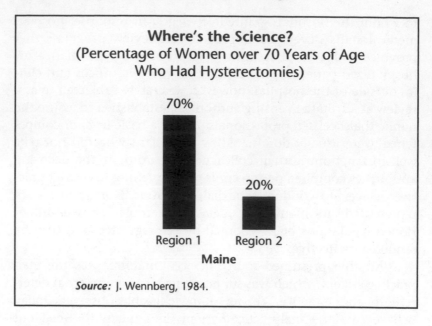

Where's the Science?
(Percentage of Women over 70 Years of Age
Who Had Hysterectomies)

70%

20%

Region 1   Region 2
Maine

Source: J. Wennberg, 1984.

1970s, Dartmouth Medical School professor John Wennberg
pioneered a series of ground-breaking studies that demonstrated huge variations in the courses of treatment doctors
around the country pursued for seemingly straightforward medical problems. He found that medicine is practiced very differently region by region, county by county, and doctor by doctor.

For example, in his earliest studies, Wennberg found that
70 percent of seventy-year-old women in one part of Maine had
received a hysterectomy, while in another geographically comparable area, only 20 percent had received one. In Iowa, the
chances that a state resident who had reached age eighty-five
had undergone a prostatectomy ranged from a low of 15 percent
to a high of more than 60 percent in other hospital markets. In
Vermont, the probability of children having a tonsillectomy
ranged from 8 percent to 70 percent (Wennberg, 1984).

Of greater interest to health insurance purchasers, similar
variations were found with respect to health care spending.
Wennberg discovered that in 1978, the average resident of New
Haven, Connecticut, consumed $215 worth of health care,

while in Boston, annual per capita health care spending averaged $448.

Although doctors like to explain away even dramatic performance variations by arguing that their patients are sicker, poorer, or more demanding than those seen by other doctors, Wennberg found that observed variations could not be explained away by underlying differences in the health of the populations or by any other obvious factor. This new knowledge had large implications. Many seized on the data as a cost-containment gold mine; it seemed that vast amounts of excessive care could be safely eliminated.

More fundamentally, Wennberg's data, supported by other researchers, undermined a fundamental attribute of professionalism, namely, that doctors practice in accordance with evidence-based standards. Most students of health care accept that medicine is not an exact science and that physicians have different styles and approaches to certain aspects of their care. But few accepted that the "art of medicine" justified the kind of practice variations that Wennberg and other researchers uncovered. Deference to professionalism suffered further from a series of studies in the 1980s that looked at whether certain surgeries, tests, and procedures were "appropriate," that is, justifiable, based on evidence from the medical literature and the expert judgment from respected practitioners in the relevant fields being studied. Researchers found that between 17 and 32 percent of the procedures studied were not performed in accordance with those objective standards (Chassin and others, 1987).

Practice variations affect both cost and quality and have not disappeared. For example, a 1995 study conducted by Harvard Medical School researchers found that after heart attacks, Medicare patients in Texas hospitals had a 50 percent greater chance of undergoing coronary angiography, an invasive dye procedure to see if coronary arteries are blocked, than did a comparable group of patients in New York hospitals. Yet over a follow-up, two-year period, many more of the Texas patients died or suffered from angina. The investigators suggested that the reason may be related to the fact that New York physicians are more likely to treat heart attack patients with life-extending beta-blocker therapy than are physicians in Texas. In short, more Texans were receiving invasive, possibly dangerous angiograms but not life-extending medication (Guadagnoli and others, 1995; Ayanian and others, 1994).

THE INFORMATION EXPLOSION

Years ago, everything most physicians needed to care for their patients was found either in their own head or in their black doctor's bag. But today, even the most conscientious, dedicated professionals cannot work effectively in isolation. They need ready access to other professionals, specialized equipment, and the most current medical information. What we know about the best medical care possible changes so often that the old methods of continuing education, like "keeping up with the literature," are no longer sufficient. These information gaps have real consequences for patients. Barely a month goes by now without a major study demonstrating important deficiencies in medical care and concluding that the fault was that physicians simply did not know better. For example, the heart attack study cited earlier revealed that about 20 percent of surveyed internists and family physicians simply were not aware of the studies on the merits of beta blockers after heart attacks. Many doctors still do not know that asthma is now considered an inflammatory disease and should be treated with inhaled steroids or that recurrent peptic ulcers have been shown to be caused by a bacteria that can be successfully treated with antibiotics. Even if they conscientiously tried to keep up with the literature, many physicians would fail to properly incorporate the newest information into their practice because most of them have never even been taught how to analyze the validity of the published studies and assimilate them into their own work (Chassin, 1996).

Computers are one obvious, potential remedy to the information glut. But, as a cottage industry, medicine was late in joining the information revolution that has swept through many other sectors of economic and social life. Electronic medical records and software that suggest courses of treatment based on volumes of medical literature are being developed and installed around the United States, but it has been a slow and difficult process and one that many physicians resist.

Paradoxically, if physicians have been slow to accept the health care information infrastructure, many patients have not. Through the Internet, as well as through television and the press, patients and their families are turning to the latest scientific journals in efforts to influence their own course of care. The information technology that physicians need to help control the blizzard of scientific developments is not simply restricted to physicians. The result has been that many patients are no longer dependent upon their physicians for sophisticated information.

TOLERANCE OF ERRORS

While we might conceivably forgive doctors for failing to keep up with rapidly changing medical literature or for practicing medicine in accordance with the norms of the communities where they learned to be doctors, the record of preventable medical mistakes is impossible to excuse. The Harvard Medical Practice Study reviewed thousands of case records from 1984 in New York State (long before there was any appreciable impact from managed care) and demonstrated that in 1 out of 100 hospitalizations, patients were injured or died as the result of what physician reviewers thought to be overt clinical negligence (Brennan and others, 1991). As graphically posed by Harvard Medical School professor Lucian Leape, as many people die in the hospital from preventable errors each year in the United States as would die if three jumbo jets crashed every two days. Imagine the public outrage, congressional hearings, and lawsuits that would result from airplanes crashing around us daily.

Such calamities do not happen because airlines, and other industries, have built vigilant and systematic approaches to reducing the possibility of mishaps. These systems assume that, despite the best efforts and intentions of highly trained individuals, human and technological mistakes are inevitable. They build-in backup systems to detect and correct mistakes before they actually compromise safety. In contrast, traditional medicine assumed that quality and safety were assured by the extraordinary efforts of individual professionals. It falsely assumed that dedicated, competent professionals should not make mistakes. It was a punitive model that presumed health professionals who committed errors should be scolded—or sued—so that they would do better next time.

The problem with this reasoning is that health care delivery is getting more, not less, complicated, and the margin for error in modern medicine has been shrinking rapidly. There has recently been a spate of stories about serious mistakes in the dispensing of medication. While the public focused on the tragic story of journalist Betsy Lehman who died at the world-renowned Dana Farber Cancer Institute in Boston of a medication error, recent studies have confirmed that, in fact, many hospitalized patients are harmed by avoidable adverse effects of drugs. Administering the wrong dose of a drug, a problem comparable to a mistake that would simply not be tolerated in many other industries, was the most common error, accounting for more than a quarter of all drug errors (Bates and others, 1997). Most of these errors did not originate with a few ignorant physicians or uncaring nurses. Rather, they were committed because of poor communication and "hand-offs" of patients among the many physicians, order transcribers, pharmacists, and nurses who work in the stressful, chaotic environment that is the modern hospital. The implication from the studies is that crucial information on dosing should be available at critical stages of the process and that monitoring for dosing errors should be greatly improved, probably through the use of computerized systems.

For purposes of this discussion, the key point is that high-quality health care no longer can be assured by the best efforts of dedicated individuals. Yet, grounded in the independence that is a cornerstone of professionalism, many physicians and other health care professionals have resisted approaches to improving quality that infringe on their autonomy, even if harmful mistakes might be reduced by adopting them.

Of course, the comparison between health care and air travel is less than perfect. Highly intensive medical interventions necessarily will result in some unanticipated and unavoidable mishaps. Much in health care cannot be reduced to the routine checks of airplane safety. Yet, like the provision of health care, safely flying an airplane is a demanding, stressful activity that relies on highly trained individuals dedicated to their jobs. Nevertheless, the airline industry assumes that pilots, mechanics, and other skilled employees will still make mistakes. Thus, it has designed and implemented safety systems that keep small errors contained. In contrast, the American health care system has generally exhibited an inability to find and define error, and when it has done so, the purpose has been more to assign blame than to fix faulty systems of care.

TOO MUCH FOCUS ON DISEASE, NOT ENOUGH ON HEALTH

The orientation of medical education, the reimbursement systems that physicians developed for themselves, and the kind of peer review that physicians conducted all support a goal of diagnosing and treating disease, and most physicians attack disease with dedication and skill. Yet, by the 1970s patients had begun to express broader goals for medicine. It was at this time that the concept of "health care" began to replace the dominant term "medical care." Today, many patients want more than skilled intervention when they are ill. They are also interested in preserving their health and, more generally, in feeling better. Many physicians were skilled at tackling major diseases, but not at providing practical advice on coping with a problem that helped a patient get through the day.

Until recently, medical education did not emphasize prevention or helping patients feel better. Furthermore, conventional health insurance usually did not pay for preventive health services that physicians and other clinicians might have provided such as nutrition counseling, cancer screening, and pain management. This is all changing now with the emergence of HMOs and heightened consumer demand, but physicians have been slow to respond to changing patient demands. One result is that patients make more visits to practitioners of alternative medical therapies, such as chiropractors and naturopaths, than to primary care physicians (Eisenberg and others, 1993).

The medical profession's seemingly single-minded dedication to attacking illness rather than promoting health also was grounded in a paternalism that by the 1970s had become unacceptable to many. In fact, the distrust of physician motivations and manner became so strong that a variety of legal safeguards emerged that were aimed at limiting professional autonomy and power. (Not until 1957 did patients even have the right to provide "informed consent" for procedures with potentially serious consequences, including death or disfigurement [Katz, 1984].)

Until the 1970s, it was common, even ethically proper, for physicians to withhold accurate prognoses from patients and their families, under the assumption that they were not emotionally equipped to handle distressing information. By the standards of just two decades later, the notion that the doctor knows best—even whether to provide accurate information based on a patient's psychological frame of mind—has become unacceptable. In a direct challenge to the long-standing underpinnings of professionalism, many patients now desire a much greater degree of personal autonomy and activism in improving their own health. In this new order, physicians still obviously play a crucial role, but they may be as focused on empowering the patient as on fighting a particular disease.

WHAT ROLE FOR PROFESSIONALISM?

The cottage industry model that dominated the practice of medicine until recent years simply was not able to adapt to the changing times. Societal forces placed greater emphasis on personal autonomy and wellness. Economic forces began to demand real value from the health care system that just was not there in the past. The challenge for the health system has changed fundamentally.

Certainly in a new model of health care delivery there still needs to be a major role for skilled individual physicians and/or other clinicians who solve problems. Nevertheless, the professional model of health care delivery is long outdated. It ignores costs, and as our population ages, that becomes more and more irresponsible. In addition, the professional model is not up to the challenge of improving quality. Centered around the endeavors of individuals, the system has tolerated avoidable errors that seriously affect patient well-being; protected physician autonomy, whether or not that autonomy is earned; shielded doctors from reasonable oversight and accountability; and focused too much on professionally adopted standards of care, even when those standards do nothing to actually improve the health and well-being of the population dependent upon the health system.

At the same time, even ardent proponents of managed care acknowledge that neither the market nor the organizations that compete in it provide an adequate substitute for the doctor-patient relationship grounded in professionalism. As one HMO Medical Director put it, "The concept of trust revolves around the physician/patient relationship rather than the institutions that surround that relationship" (Newcomer, 1997).

Nevertheless, in important ways, managed care seeks to change the nature of medical professionalism. In particular, managed care organizations want to substitute ongoing monitoring and judgment of competence for the limited peer review of professional organizations. In line with emerging consumer attitudes, the best of them want to expand the goals of medicine beyond a single-minded attack on illness to include attention to broader concepts of health and well-being. And, as we will discuss, they seek to substitute the concept of value—quality at a reasonable cost—for quality at any cost.

In some ways, then, managed care seeks to have its cake and eat it too. It wants to substitute itself for aspects of professionalism that have not worked very well and that it wishes to repudiate. But it also assumes that the core principle of professionalism—a doctor-patient relationship based on trust—will emerge unscarred by the rest of what managed care brings with it. In other words, managed care proponents expect—perhaps, hope—that physicians will both want and be able to act in the best interests of their patients even as managed care shifts much of the flow of dollars and the running of the delivery system from physicians to mostly for-profit corporations.

In fact, as we will discuss in Chapter 6, physicians and patients often feel that managed care has actually run roughshod over the doctor-patient relationship. For now, we turn to the evolution of managed care and how it has attempted to address the failings of the professional model.

3

The Rise of Managed Care | *Birth of the Blues*

Today many people see managed care organizations as modern corporate behemoths, often more responsive to shareholders than to patient needs. But managed care, especially in the HMO form, is much older and more rooted in idealism than people generally appreciate. In fact, the direct forerunners of today's HMOs were founded in the 1930s by physicians disgruntled with traditional practice. Some, especially those in rural areas, were organized as consumer cooperatives. In 1929, Dr. Michael Shadid formed a rural cooperative in which participating farmers each purchased $50 shares to raise capital for a new hospital, receiving discounted medical care in return. (His efforts would almost cost him his license to practice medicine and did cost him his membership in the county medical society [Fox, 1966].) In urban areas, subscribers and supporters included liberal and even socialist representatives of business, labor, the medical profession, and government (Starr, 1982).

The core of the new concept was the so-called prepaid group practice, an aggregation of physicians that emphasized preventive medicine and formal consumer representation in the organization's governance. For a single payment per month, members were entitled to medical care without extra charges as long as they sought care from physicians working in the medical group. Rooted as they were in political populism, these health plans were strictly nonprofit.

In the forties, the more successful prepaid group practices expanded in urban centers. Kaiser Permanente achieved a foothold in parts of the West Coast, as did Group Health Cooperative of Puget Sound in Seattle, Health Insurance Plan (HIP) in

New York, and Group Health Association in Washington, D.C. These organizations survived and even thrived primarily because they were able to provide more comprehensive health coverage with little of the out-of-pocket payments that traditional insurance required of patients. Interestingly, these forerunners of present-day HMOs did not offer lower premiums than traditional insurance. Rather, many employees picked them because of the financial security they offered or because they were attracted to the group practice model of health delivery, in which most medical care was delivered under one roof.

EARLY OPPOSITION

From the beginning, managed care faced vigorous opposition, not from consumers or aggrieved employees, but from organized medicine. Most doctors, and especially their organizations, viewed the new arrangements as threatening to the conventional fee-for-service system and their dominant role in it, and they expended considerable energy to keep prepaid group practice on the fringes of health care delivery. In some communities, medical societies attacked the concept as "socialism." Physicians practicing in the groups were intimidated and victimized by the anticompetitive behavior of other doctors. Physician organizers of prepaid groups often were expelled by their local medical societies and even ostracized socially (Starr, 1982).

In one prominent case, the American Medical Association tried to destroy the Group Health Association (GHA), a consumer cooperative in Washington, D.C. The AMA first attempted to persuade legal authorities to take action against what it regarded as "unlicensed, unregulated health insurance and the corporate practice of medicine." When that route of attack failed, the AMA and the local medical society threatened reprisals against doctors who worked for the group, prevented them from obtaining consultations and referrals, and persuaded every hospital in the District of Columbia to deny GHA physicians admitting privileges. This last move effectively cut off GHA members from hospital care.

In 1943, the Supreme Court agreed that the AMA had violated antitrust laws by conspiring against the cooperative, and GHA survived. But the efforts of organized medicine put many other fledgling group practices out of business. Facing professional isolation, few physicians were willing to participate. And many state legislatures buckled under pressure from medical societies, passing laws that required all insurance plans to allow free choice of physicians, effectively banning the HMO approach.

Despite these efforts to undermine them, by the fifties prepaid group practices, such as Kaiser and HIP, had established particular niches in a few, mostly urban, communities. But they were not an important force in American medicine. Organized medicine had been so successful at limiting their growth that it no longer had to engage in anticompetitive behavior directed against them. Because private practitioners were not willing to participate in them, prepaid plans would have had to establish their own facilities, an expensive proposition.

Besides, in the 1950s and the first part of the 1960s, health care costs were not a major societal or economic problem. Commercial insurers, especially Blue Cross and Blue Shield plans, were willing and able to offer conventional insurance that accepted the control of medical professionals over health delivery. Indeed, the Blues originally had been set up by providers to efficiently pay claims for services rendered.

For most of their early history, then, prepaid health plans had little effect on the dominant health care system. They appealed to a limited number individuals who preferred the group practice style, the comprehensive benefits, and the protection from out-of-pocket expenses that conventional insurers charged. But outside of the limelight, they were establishing a significant beachhead and offering an alternative to a system that would soon implode.

THE 1970s AND THE HEALTH MAINTENANCE ORGANIZATION

Ironically, the "alternative" prepaid group practice movement would get a lift from the conservative Nixon Administration.

Health officials under Nixon were influenced by managed care's first real intellectual leaders and visionaries, especially an iconoclastic pediatric neurologist from Minnesota named Paul Ellwood, who coined the term "health maintenance organization" (HMO). The label was an attempt to recognize the new financial incentives and commitment to comprehensive care that prepaid group practices offered. Nixon Administration health officials thought HMOs had the potential to lower health care costs. Largely because HMOs relied on private-sector initiative rather than a new government bureaucracy, the Republican administration embraced the HMO concept.

In early 1971, President Nixon announced a new national health strategy based on the expansion of HMOs, predicting that by the end of the decade there would be 1,300 HMOs caring for at least 65 million people. The centerpiece of the Nixon program was the HMO Act of 1973, which provided start-up grants and loans for HMOs. As a further spur to HMO development, the act also required large employers to offer their employees the option of at least one HMO, where one was available. Given their roots in consumerism and the labor movement, expansion of prepaid group practices was endorsed by Democrats as well as by the Nixon Administration, and the act passed with bipartisan support.

But the Nixon Administration's optimistic projections about managed care growth would prove to be off by almost twenty years. In 1981, there were only about 300 HMO plans serving 10 million enrollees. As a result of their limited growth, prepaid group practices had little impact on the fee-for-service sector in which most physicians operated. They were two systems of health care operating separately. Over time, the medical profession even learned to tolerate prepaid group practices in the few communities where they operated. It would be almost another decade before employer purchasers began to see HMOs as their only practical alternative to the problem of spiraling health care premiums. Only then would prepaid groups become a real threat to mainstream medicine.

THE RISE OF HMOs AND THE
LOSS OF PHYSICIAN DOMINATION

By the mid-1980s, the forces described in Chapters 1 and 2 had conspired to drive health care costs inexorably upward. At some point, purchasers of health care would take no more. That breaking point occurred in the mid-to-late 1980s, when employers began to decide they could no longer tolerate the costs of the conventional indemnity insurance system, that government could not effectively deal with the cost problem, and that managed care, and HMOs especially, might provide a viable alternative.

As enrollment began to rise sharply (an average of more than 20 percent per year between 1983 and 1986 [Millenson, 1997b]), managed care plans in some regions began to accumulate market power and achieve new leverage over providers that was never possible under traditional insurance. The essence of that leverage was the threat of moving business (i.e., patients) elsewhere, and it became credible for two primary reasons. First, unlike traditional insurers, managed care organizations (MCOs) had control over the "covered lives" in their plans; they could channel patients to doctors with whom they had contracts. Thus, providers not in a network would lose access to whole blocks of patients—including their own former patients. Additionally, the widespread excess of health delivery capacity in most urban and suburban communities meant that managed care organizations could afford both to exclude many providers and demand that those who signed up accept lower prices. Gradually, the health care marketplace began to look like other marketplaces. An excess of supply meant that prices would come down.

Discounting was not the only way managed care pulled down health care costs. Plans launched "preauthorization programs" that required patients and their physicians to seek plan approval for high-cost services, including admission to a hospital. MCOs also prodded doctors and hospitals to move as much

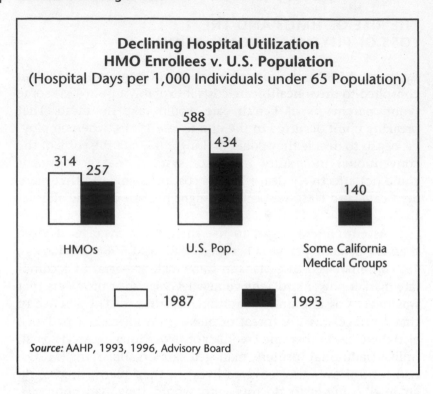

Declining Hospital Utilization
HMO Enrollees v. U.S. Population
(Hospital Days per 1,000 Individuals under 65 Population)

588
434
314 257
140

HMOs   U.S. Pop.   Some California
                                  Medical Groups

[ ] 1987   ■ 1993

Source: AAHP, 1993, 1996, Advisory Board

care as possible from inpatient to outpatient settings. Between 1987 and 1993, HMO hospitalization rates, as measured by number of days spent in the hospital per 1,000 plan members dropped from 314 a year to 257 for the under-65 population. The comparable numbers for all insurance plans were 588 and 434, respectively (Gabel, 1993; 1996). Referrals to technology-oriented, highly paid specialists declined as well. As the 1990s approached, and as proof of managed care's capacity to lower costs grew more evident, employers' reliance on managed care snowballed.

Then, at some point in the early 1990s, employers began to realize that they were only riding on the managed care bandwagon, when they could be driving. Just as managed care organizations had demanded lower fees from providers, employers began to demand lower premiums from managed care organizations. In effect, they began to demand that managed care plans stop pricing themselves just below fee-for-service plans, a practice economists call "shadow pricing," and start actually competing with each other.

This more aggressive form of competition led, in turn, to rapid changes in some markets and still more cost cutting. The revolution we are now experiencing was under way. In the space of just a few years, price competition had entered health care. Although physicians and some health economists argued that managed care's success in holding down costs simply reflected its enrollment of a healthier population that needed fewer services, the continued cost-cutting success of HMOs overpowered these theoretical and fairly technical arguments. It was easy to measure the purchasers' bottom lines, managed care saved them money.

Between 1981 and 1985, even with the HMO Act no longer in effect, the number of HMO enrollees had almost doubled. By 1988, enrollment stood at almost 33 million, and in 1995, at 56 million. By 1998, it had reached approximately 80 million,[1] and with increasing numbers of Medicaid and Medicare enrollees moving into managed care plans, projections for the year 2000 are in the neighborhood of 100 million.

MANAGED CARE DIVERSIFIES

For most of its early life, managed care suffered from limited appeal, largely because it only came in one flavor. As discussed earlier, the first HMOs were outgrowths of prepaid group practices that developed as distinct delivery systems with their own exclusive doctors, and in the case of Kaiser Permanente and HIP, even with their own hospitals. Patients joining an HMO entered a completely separate system for their health care. For some, particularly the young and healthy and those who had grown

---

1. Surveys vary here, largely depending on whether (1) point-of-service (POS) plans are counted as HMOs and (2) whether Medicare and Medicaid beneficiaries are included. The 80 million figure used here includes most enrollees in POS plans (some are actually in preferred provider organizations) and all HMO enrollees in Medicare and Medicaid.

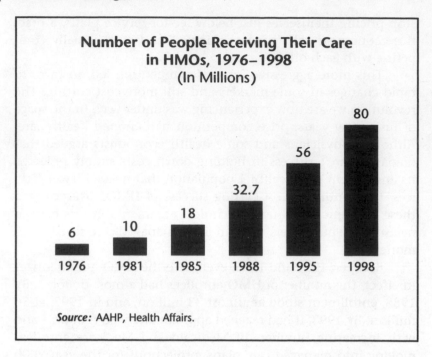

Number of People Receiving Their Care in HMOs, 1976–1998
(In Millions)

Year	Value
1976	6
1981	10
1985	18
1988	32.7
1995	56
1998	80

Source: AAHP, Health Affairs.

up in these programs, the alternative was appealing. But for many individuals who had ties to personal physicians or who were more comfortable visiting traditional solo or small group practices, care in a "clinic" was unacceptable and they resisted the change.

But during the 1980s, new HMOs began competing with the traditional prepaid group practices by contracting with networks of private physicians called independent practice associations (IPAs). In this newer form of HMO, physicians provide care for HMO patients in their own offices, not a shared clinic. This model kept health plans from having to invest in "bricks and mortar," or hire their own personnel. The IPA approach also enabled HMOs to enter new markets more quickly and with much lower capital expenses than had the traditional prepaid group practices.

Most important, in distinct contrast to prepaid group practices, the IPA approach permitted physicians to contract with many managed care organizations at the same time. Under such arrangements, physicians could also maintain their own practices. As for patients, they could have a much wider choice of physician than was generally offered by prepaid group practices. And employers enjoyed lower premiums than under traditional insurance, although perhaps not as low as under the group practice model. Very quickly, the IPA emerged as the fastest growing form of HMO. Between 1989 and 1994, the percentage of HMO enrollees in IPA or network HMOs rose from 58 to 69 percent, while the percentage of enrollees in more traditional staff and group models fell from 42 to 32 percent. By the early 1990s, nearly two-thirds of total HMO growth was in IPA plans (Zelman, 1996).

NEW NICHES AND NEW PRODUCTS

The rise of managed care has been much more than the rise and evolution of traditional or IPA-model HMOs. It has also been defined by the growth of preferred provider organizations (PPOs), which apply managed care tools in a fee-for-service format, and by the emergence of a new product, the point-of-service (POS) plan, which combines elements of the HMO with elements of the old full-choice system. By offering less restrictive options—that is, more physician choice—and in the case of the PPO, an option that meshed with the needs of self-insuring employers, these approaches to managed care have been critical to its ascendancy.

For many employers and individuals, HMOs, with their closed provider networks, were too restrictive. PPOs placed more moderate restrictions on patient choice. For example, in a typical PPO insurance product, patients generally pay 20 to 30 percent of the charge for going outside of the contracted network of providers, whereas a patient going out of network in an HMO has to pay the entire bill.

In addition to providing more choice of provider, PPOs offer some employers another major advantage over HMOs. Due to details of insurance law, which we will discuss later, PPOs (but not HMOs) are very compatible with self-insurance. When self-insuring, employers technically do not purchase

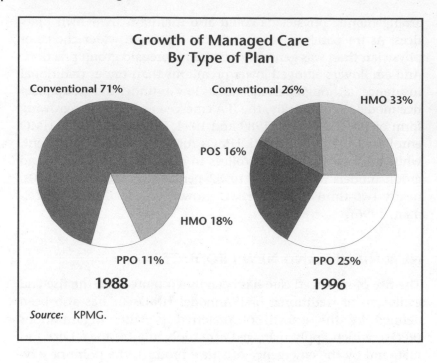

**Growth of Managed Care
By Type of Plan**

Conventional 71%

POS 16%

HMO 18%

PPO 11%

1988

Conventional 26%

HMO 33%

PPO 25%

1996

Source: KPMG.

health insurance at all. Instead, they set aside a pool of funds and directly pay their employees' medical bills. The advantage, as many employers see it, is the freedom from state insurance regulation that often mandates specific benefits or imposes consumer protection procedures that generally increase the cost of coverage. The downside is that self-insurers are usually limited to using PPO products. And since PPOs still employ the fee-for-service payment mechanism, they are able to use only some of the management tools that HMOs typically employ. Not surprisingly, purchasers have found that their costs for PPO care have fallen between those of traditional insurance and a tightly run HMO.

Many health care analysts thought PPOs would serve as a transition from traditional insurance to HMOs. It was widely assumed that they would wither away as HMOs proved more cost effective and as employees came to accept the new restrictions. But because of their attractiveness to self-insuring employers and their compatibility with the public's demand for choice of doctor, they have not only survived but actually flourished. Enrollment increases in PPOs have equalled those in HMOs, moving from 28 million in 1987 to somewhere between 70 and 80 million in 1996.[2] Over time, by adopting some managed care techniques used by HMOs, PPOs have been able to keep costs down, at least compared to conventional insurance plans. Moreover, since many of a PPO's additional costs—specifically, deductibles and co-insurance—are paid by patients themselves, PPOs remain relatively inexpensive to the employer.

In the 1990s, health plans developed still another product to help employers bridge the gap between the cost savings associated with HMOs and the broader choice of providers used in traditional insurance and PPO products. In increasing numbers, HMOs offered a "point of service" (POS) option, which allows HMO members to go out of network whenever they choose and pay a specified co-insurance amount out of their own pocket. In its use of financial incentives for patients to receive care in the designated network of providers, the POS option resembles a PPO. The main difference is that the in-network care generally takes place in an HMO's cost-control environment, including the use of gatekeepers and capped payments to physicians.

For employers willing to give up the benefits of self-insurance, the POS option offers considerable appeal. Because it produces most of the cost savings associated with HMOs while preserving the safety valve for members to have a broader choice of providers, POS has been the fastest growing managed care product in recent years. Today, over 75 percent of HMOs offer a POS option, (Dial and others, 1996) and perhaps 20 percent of Americans with employer-based insurance are in plans with a POS option, an increase from just 4 to 5 percent a few years ago.[3]

---

2. Figures on the number of enrollees in PPOs are notoriously unreliable, largely due to problems of definition and to the greater difficulty of getting accurate numbers on self-insured plans.

3. Estimates of POS enrollment vary considerably, depending on definitions applied.

FROM MINORITY TO MAJORITY STATUS

Through traditional HMOs, IPA-HMOs, PPOs, POS plans and their variations, managed care now offers purchasers a wide variety of options. For those purchasers most concerned about cost, there are plenty of tightly managed HMOs around, many offering reasonably broad networks of private physicians whom their employees already see. For those employers who think HMOs offer too little choice of provider, the POS variant provides a kind of relief valve. For those who want to avoid state insurance regulation, or who want a product that looks more like traditional insurance, PPOs are widespread and increasingly use many of the cost-containing techniques associated with HMOs.

Moreover, employers do not have to choose among many plans to offer their workers these options. Most MCOs now offer a menu of products, so employers can pick one insurer and get a variety of choices, thereby substituting choice *within* a plan for choice *among* plans. Moreover, because the POS option provides an opportunity for a covered employee to go to any provider, albeit by paying for the privilege, many employers no longer feel the need to accommodate employee demands for access to their own physicians by offering a choice of plans. The POS option can satisfy the any-and-every-physician requirement.

As managed care approaches the end of the twentieth century, the preferred product appears to be a hybrid plan—essentially an IPA-type HMO, with a wide choice of individual physicians or groups, that still offers a point-of-service relief valve. That evolution, it appears, has been driven by a continuing concern, experienced by many employees and probably fueled by physicians, that more traditional HMO arrangements place too many restrictions on choice of physician. But as we will discuss in detail in Chapter 8, the growing acceptance of approaches that permit subscribers a broad choice of physicians and other providers may have the perverse effect of undermining the organizational benefits of integrated group practice, the innovation that led to HMOs in the first place. We will find that managed care's more recent evolution is a story of a good idea going potentially astray by trying to be more like the system it once sought to replace.

Whatever the specific future of managed care, in choosing between the multiple managed care options, increasing numbers of employers were making one common decision: to abandon the conventional insurance plans that were the dominant form of insurance entering the 1980s. Even small employers, many of whom had continued throughout the 1980s to offer mostly traditional insurance plans, had begun switching to managed care. As many analysts concluded, "Managed care isn't coming; it has arrived" (Jensen, 1997).

THE TRENDS CONVERGE

During the late 1980s and early 1990s, the trends emerging in the managed care marketplace converged with employer frustration over soaring health care costs. The result was predictable, even inevitable. Enrollment in HMOs and PPOs of various forms soared.

The public sector, equally concerned about costs, would not be far behind. In the mid-1990s, state and federal governments undertook a series of steps to move—in some cases almost overnight—large numbers of Medicaid and Medicare recipients into managed care, mostly HMOs. Because many states required Medicaid recipients to enroll in HMOs, between 1993 and 1997 the numbers of Medicaid recipients in managed care leaped from 3.6 million to approximately 15 million (Medicaid Facts, 1996).[4] Further increases were on state administrative drawing boards. Enrollment in Medicare managed care plans lagged behind largely because participation by Medicare beneficiaries in HMOs remained elective.

But here too, rapid change was the order of the day. Between 1993 and 1997 the number of Medicare beneficiaries in managed care plans rose from 2.6 to about 5 million ("The Medicare Program," 1997), with estimates of managed care

---

4. Due to rapidly changing enrollment in the states, 1997 numbers are estimates only.

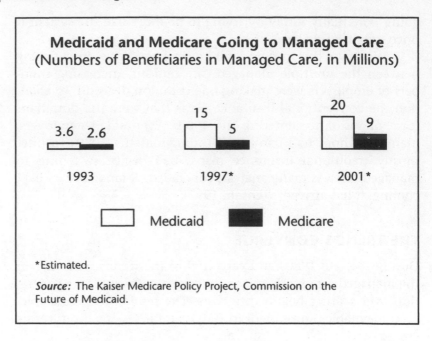

Medicaid and Medicare Going to Managed Care
(Numbers of Beneficiaries in Managed Care, in Millions)

20

15

3.6 2.6   5   9

1993   1997*   2001*

☐ Medicaid   ■ Medicare

*Estimated.

Source: The Kaiser Medicare Policy Project, Commission on the Future of Medicaid.

enrollment in 2001 reaching 9 million or more. (Medicare restructuring passed as part of the 1997 Balanced Budget Act, will only hasten the trend.) And given the high premiums paid by Medicare for senior citizens in managed care plans, competition for Medicare enrollments among managed care plans in many communities was intense, to say the least. Overall, the public-sector movement toward managed care was so swift and significant that by the mid-1990s, many analysts viewed Medicaid and Medicare as the biggest drivers of marketplace change.

THE CLINTON PLAN: MANAGED CARE AND MARKETS EMERGE VICTORIOUS

President Clinton's health care reform proposal would confirm and ratify the victory of managed care. Reform supporters would promise over and over again that the President's plan would not eliminate the cherished insurance arrangement in which individuals had full choice of provider. In fact, in an effort to allay such fears, the Clinton plan would actually have guaranteed access to such arrangements, an access that had already disappeared for millions.

But the Clinton plan also envisioned a changing health care marketplace in which price competition among managed care health plans would be the rule of the day. Such competition, it was widely assumed, would produce the proverbial nail in the coffin of the traditional insurance system. Simply put, it would not be able to compete.

Additionally, although many would not see it, the Clinton plan also signaled an important milestone in the debate over whether competition or regulation should drive health care change. The scope and magnitude of change proposed in the Clinton plan would produce an image, sometimes reflecting reality, of widespread government intervention. In so doing, the plan offered up the specter of big government that would eventually be used to kill it.

Still, it would be an ironic death. For all its "big government" accouterments, the Clinton plan was actually based on the expectation that marketplace competition—specifically, competition among managed care plans—and not government regulation should and would be the driving force behind health system change.

In these ways the Clinton plan, for all its failings, represented both an affirmation of the recent past and an accurate prediction of the immediate future. Managed care would be the engine of change, and market competition would be the fuel.

4

The Tools of Managed Care

You Can't Always Get What You Want

Earlier in this book, we reviewed why the fee-for-service system of health care financing and delivery in the United States was flawed and bound for failure. It neither constrained costs nor promoted health care quality. It was a system that allowed costs to be shifted around and passed on until almost no one knew what they were paying for health care. As a result, we all paid far more than we likely would have if we had faced normal market pressures and constraints. The old system also gave physicians almost complete autonomy in the practice of medicine, a value that seems unassailable until one looks more deeply into its problems: fragmented care, doctors who are unable to keep up with clinical advances, and the profligate incentives of a system that pays by the procedure.

In Chapter 3, we saw how attractive managed care looked to the people paying the bills—the nation's businesses and government. They turned to managed care largely as a last resort and sometimes, in the case of businesses, against the wishes of their employees. Thus, the story we have told so far has been largely one of economics and money. But there is, of course, significantly more to it than that. Managed care organizations claim to be much more than cost-reduction machines. The name "managed care" implies that it will bring order, coordination, and rationality to the care process. But how is it supposed to do that? And has it worked? Those are the questions we turn to now.

THE LOGIC OF MANAGED CARE

A steady drumbeat of media criticism often suggests that all managed care works pretty much the same way. Nothing could be farther from the truth. Organizations tailor everything from their marketing posture to their relationships with doctors to fit what they think purchasers and consumers in their local markets will want and to what they think will turn a profit. Moreover, the shape of managed care changes and evolves, often in ever faster cycles. Even if we attempted here to catalog every type of managed care arrangement in the marketplace today, the list would be incomplete and out-of-date by the time this book was published. Analysts are always pointing to trends, and many confidently predict which types of plans or arrangements will predominate in the immediate future. But, as often as not, they're wrong.

Today, if one trend stands out, it is hybridization. HMOs used to be classified into four types or models, known as staff, group, network, and independent practice association (IPA). The classifications were based on the nature of the relationships between the insurer/HMO and physicians. But in recent years, these categories have become less useful, and sometimes even misleading. Today, most HMO plans are likely to be a mix of one or more of the models. And any one insurer may operate several different hybrids in different markets—even in the same market.

Plans also vary by how they operate, the strategies they employ, and the tools they use. Some health plans carefully manage the activities of their providers and assume an active role in the management and organization of health care delivery. At the other end of the spectrum, many plans perform only the traditional insurance functions, leaving decision making on health care delivery and even considerable financial responsibility to providers or groups of providers. Some plans view physicians and hospitals as partners, whereas others consider them vendors with whom the plan must bargain.

Still, in a world of hybrids and variation, there are some core constants. There is a logic to managed care that finds some form of expression in almost all plans, and there are certain tools of managed care that almost all plans will employ, at least to some extent.

One way of looking at managed care is as a mirror image of the fee-for-service system. Ideally, fragmentation is replaced with organization, cost-unconsciousness with cost-consciousness, a blank check with checks and balances, and professional autonomy with accountability. Most specifically, the fee-for-service incentive to do everything possible is replaced by the incentive to keep patients healthy and to do only what may be necessary and appropriate.

The logic relies heavily on more and better communication between nurse, primary care physician, and specialist—about which of them should perform what services, about which treatments may work and which may not, about which providers might be doing too much or too little, about how to keep physicians up-to-speed, and about how to get patients more actively involved in caring for themselves. In sum, the logic of managed care assumes that the management of care will produce a more organized, more coordinated system that does a better job of both keeping costs under control and improving the health of the population to be served.

We will soon see that this theoretical logic frequently does not translate into real-world practice. But first we turn our attention to the basic types of managed care plans doing business today and the basic tools they use to organize the financing and delivery of health care.

A TAXONOMY OF MANAGED CARE

We could list an alphabet soup of managed care varieties here, but we will keep it simple. Today there are two basic forms of managed care organization: the health maintenance organization (HMO) and the preferred provider organization (PPO). (Some would list a third form called managed fee-for-sevice, in which traditional fee-for-service insurers pay bills with oversight. But managed fee-for-sevice does not include a selected provider network, a hallmark of managed care.)

Choice and Cost in Health Plan Types

	Traditional HMO Staff/ Group Models	IPA HMO	PPO	Conventional Plan
Size of Network	Limited	Larger	As in IPA	Unlimited
Right to Go Out of Network	No	No	Yes (at higher cost)	Does not apply
Cost	Lowest	Low	Higher (especially to consumer)	Highest

Note: HMOs may have a point-of-service option, which will increase cost.

An HMO is a health insurer that assumes responsibility for providing comprehensive health services to a formally enrolled population in return for a predetermined payment. HMOs come in many shapes and varieties. The traditional "group" and "staff" model HMOs still tend to contract with or employ an exclusive provider network. The newer "network" or "IPA" models contract with individual providers or groups of providers who maintain similar contractual relationships with other health plans. HMOs tend to "lock-in" patients. That is, unless they are willing to pick up the entire bill for going outside of the contracted network, HMO enrollees receive services only from contracted or employed providers. Out-of-pocket costs to enrolled members are generally very low, usually either $5 or $10 a visit. But, as discussed in Chapter 3, because many consumers object to the lock-in feature, over 75 percent of HMOs now offer a point-of-service (POS) option, which gives patients the option of seeking the care of a doctor outside of the HMO network for a price.

A PPO is a much looser arrangement than an HMO and bears more resemblance to traditional insurance, particularly in using fee-for-service payment to physicians. Patients may see any provider in the network, and pay only a modest portion of provider charges. PPO members may also see providers not in the network, but for a significantly higher out-of-pocket payment. PPOs, therefore, as noted in Chapter 3, may offer more choice of provider but generally at a higher price, especially to the consumer.

The definitions suggest perhaps two core differences that seem particularly important for our purposes here. First, in HMOs, physicians are generally under much greater pressure to control costs. In PPOs, physicians are more likely to find—as in the old system—that they make more when they do more. Second, HMOs generally involve a much tighter and more coordinated organizational structure. Among other things, this means that they may have more capacity—for better or worse—to apply the tools of managed care. It is for this reason that consumer concerns about managed care generally focus on HMOs. However, PPOs commonly use one of the managed care tools that doctors resent most, namely, utilization management programs that review and sometimes reject the clinical recommendations of physicians. As we will demonstrate in Chapter 6, HMOs are often singled out and criticized for cost-control activities also performed by PPOs and even by more traditional, full-choice insurers.

MANAGED CARE'S TOOL BOX

The tools of managed care attempt to address the deficits of fee-for-service medicine, especially its unrestrained use of services. Like the variations of styles and structures in managed care organizations, the tools may be used in an infinite combination of ways. But three of the tools described in this chapter are fundamental to managed care and can be found at some level in almost all plans, whatever their type. The fourth tool, prepayment, is central to HMOs but not PPOs.

In reviewing these tools, we should keep three points in mind. First, all the tools have a logic and potential value, but all can also be misused, to the detriment of patients. Second, all the tools have components aimed *both* at controlling costs and at

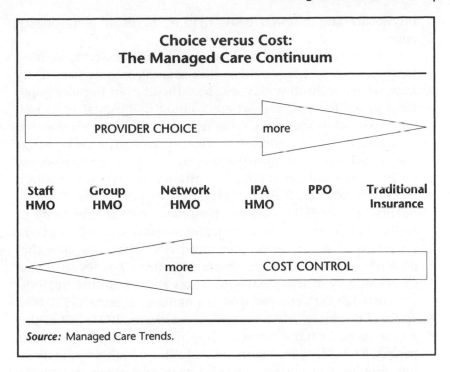

Choice versus Cost:
The Managed Care Continuum

PROVIDER CHOICE   more

| Staff | Group | Network | IPA | PPO | Traditional |
| HMO | HMO | HMO | HMO | | Insurance |

more   COST CONTROL

Source: Managed Care Trends.

improving quality. Third, the elements of the tools aimed at managing quality are more recent, less well developed, and often neglected, relative to those aimed at controlling cost. As a result, most managed care organizations have been far more successful in efforts to control costs than in efforts to improve quality. We shall return to this third point later on.

Selective Contracting

Selection of network physicians is, we believe, the feature that most defines managed care and distinguishes it from conventional fee-for-service plans. Selective contracting, as it is called, offers an antidote to many of the core problems of fee-for-service plans. To control costs, a health plan that selectively contracts can use the threat of *not* contracting to achieve more favorable payment rates with providers. That threat is particularly effective in areas where there are too many specialist physicians and hospital beds, that is, in most metropolitan areas.

But there are limits to this strategy. In some communities, there may be so few providers that excluding some is virtually impossible. Exclusions may also be difficult even in more populated areas, for example, where a clinic or hospital is so well regarded that its inclusion in the network is a practical necessity.

Selective contracting also affords managed care networks the opportunity to improve quality by selecting providers based on their skill and reputation. For instance, in certain specialized areas of medicine, like coronary artery bypass grafts (CABGs), quality is related to volume. Hospitals that do hundreds of CABGs per year generally have faster recoveries, and fewer complications, and may even offer lower costs than hospitals that do a few per month. For example, one study has revealed that CABG surgery at the prestigious Texas Heart Institute in Houston costs $26,000, compared with a national average of $30,000, and still produces better outcomes (Pearlstein, 1997). All of this is consistent with the commonsense notion that practice makes perfect. The ability to steer patients to those high-volume facilities should be a critical part of a managed care's strategy to reduce costs while improving clinical care.

Not surprisingly, both providers and patients have accepted selective contracting only grudgingly. What patients see first is the loss of access to a favored physician or the inability to go to any specialist or hospital. They fear the worst; that plans will choose providers based not on their competence but on their willingness to accept the deepest discounts. Thus, patients may assume that the best providers (who patients often believe to be their own) may not be chosen to participate, and may not need to participate, in managed care.

Meanwhile, some doctors complain about being excluded from certain managed care networks, and others resent being forced to accept lower fees. At times they find themselves in a limited network with other physicians whom they do not know, or worse, whom they do know as poor-quality physicians. Doctors frequently complain that limited networks prevent them from serving their patients' best interests.

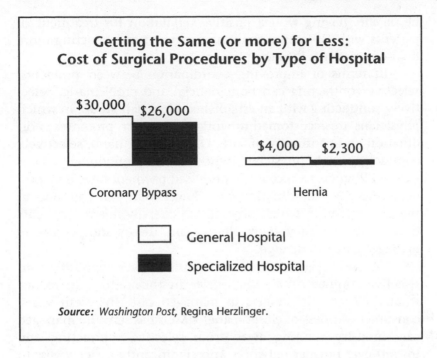

**Getting the Same (or more) for Less:
Cost of Surgical Procedures by Type of Hospital**

$30,000 $26,000

$4,000 $2,300

Coronary Bypass   Hernia

General Hospital

Specialized Hospital

Source: Washington Post, Regina Herzlinger.

Without question, there is something to this critique. To date, health plans have been much more likely to use selective contracting as a blunt instrument for achieving price discounts from financially insecure physicians than as a precision instrument for promoting coordination or building a top-notch panel of providers. However, in recent years, some managed care plans have taken selective contracting to a more sophisticated level. They have started analyzing the patient loads, diagnoses, and outcomes of their network physicians to see how they compare with their peers on performance indices, including use of services. Such "profiling" permits plans to select and adjust their roster of doctors based on objective cost-effectiveness data. Predictably, again, some physicians complain that these profiles ignore important determinants of utilization such as the underlying state of health and illness of their patients or the quality of care delivered. In a worst-case scenario, a physician might be dropped from a network because he or she, having won a positive reputation for treatment of patients with HIV disease or diabetes, was now attracting more high-cost patients into the plan.

In terms of improving coordination between providers, selective contracting can be beneficial and problematic. Selectively contracting with an established physician group, in which physicians are accustomed to working together, promotes coordination and continuity of care. On the other hand, selectively contracting with physicians whose only common ground is their willingness to accept the proposed payment rates may produce a level of coordination even lower than that common in the old system, in which physicians generally referred patients to those doctors they knew. Here, again, theory and practice of managed care can diverge.

Consumer groups have sometimes made opposition to selective contracting a *cause célèbre* in their efforts to reduce what they view as dangers in managed care. In recent years, consumer wariness of closed-panel HMOs has sent the managed care industry running away from selective contracting and toward ever broader networks and significantly easier access to "out of network" physicians, including specialists. In some markets, specialist physicians may have managed care contracts with fifty or more organizations.

But broad expansion of networks, although responsive to consumer demand, may turn out to be an ill-advised strategy. An all-physicians-in-all-networks scenario clearly undermines the power and potential value of selective contracting. Cost control can also certainly suffer, as consumer demands for broader choice strengthen the bargaining position of providers who now feel less threatened by potential exclusion. Quality, too, may suffer, as physicians contracting with multiple managed care organizations have little commitment to any of them and as managed care organizations lose the capacity to engage providers in innovative and more coordinated team approaches. As much as consumers dislike (and misunderstand) it, without selective contracting, managed care would be much less able to produce the important cost reductions it has achieved.

UTILIZATION MANAGEMENT AND
PREAUTHORIZATION

If HMOs have demonstrated anything, it is that with a relentless focus on reducing the use of unnecessary medical services, especially days spent by patients in the hospital, they can reduce health care costs. As we noted in Chapter 3, hospital utilization rates began falling in the late 1980s and continue to fall today. Many keep suggesting that these reductions must stop somewhere, but it still not clear where that point may be. In California, where managed care has, in many respects, reached its most mature state, the number of HMO hospital days per 1,000 enrollees has dropped to 230, compared to a national HMO average of 297, and a national average of all insurance plans of over 450. Some California plans or large medical groups that assume responsibility for all medical care have numbers as low as 130 (Health Care Advisory Board, 1996).

Similar evidence of cost reductions came from a wide variety of studies of different medical procedures and communities. The old system was so rife with inappropriate or unnecessary procedures, tests, and hospitalizations, that significant reductions in these activities could be achieved and without threatening quality. HMOs accomplished these objectives through an array of techniques broadly called "utilization management" (UM). Such efforts had been undertaken even by traditional insurers. But it was with HMOs that utilization management really took off.

The chief UM strategy is called "preauthorization," in which a physician's recommendation for complex or costly services is evaluated by trained HMO personnel (usually nurses). They seek to determine if the recommendation meets the plan's definition of "medically necessary" care and whether that care could be provided in a lower cost setting. If the physician request for care is approved, it is said to be "preauthorized" and will be paid for. Typically, all nonemergency hospital admissions are subject to such review, and emergency admissions must be reviewed within a short period following admission. The need for continued hospital care is assessed periodically (Gray and Field, 1989).

Utilization management, combined with advancing medical technology, sparked an explosion in outside the hospital care. Naturally, this movement of care to outpatient settings led health plans to scrutinize not only whether a particular procedure was necessary, but where—in or out of the hospital—it should be performed. Expensive outpatient procedures such as "same day" surgery in a surgicenter, MRI scans, and sleep studies might also be subject to UM. Some managed care organizations even began requiring preauthorization for routine specialty referrals from a primary care physician.

Theoretically, all services could be subjected to preauthorization requirements. But such a strategy would result in a bureaucratic nightmare. Indeed, since plans apply the preauthorization requirement in wide varieties of ways, many physicians already find UM requirements burdensome and inefficient. At their worst, physicians argue, these requirements are insulting and represent a challenge to their authority and autonomy that could result in a denial of care their patients need. Their objections invoke images of highly trained, experienced specialists being told by a review nurse 3,000 miles away: "No, we won't allow you to keep the patient you call 'critically ill' in the hospital for another day because she has not met our criteria. Send her home."

There's no doubt that such abuses occur. But, for the most part, preauthorization requirements tend to be applied to anticipated, discrete, and relatively expensive services, not to emergencies or routine medical decisions that practitioners make.

A more systemic dilemma posed by UM is the question of who becomes responsible and even legally liable when the insurer makes judgments about what is covered by insurance. What should happen when a physician believes a procedure or a test is medically indicated but the insurer determines that the particular service is either not a "covered benefit" or not "medically necessary?" Health plans typically take the legal position that they are merely making payment decisions, not practicing medicine, which, they say, should remain within the domain of practicing physicians. Doctors counter that their ability to practice medicine in the patients' best interests often hinges on a plan's willingness to pay.

Here the insurer's case is often weak. If a health plan denies coverage of a $200,000 bone marrow transplant for a breast cancer patient, and she cannot afford it herself, she will almost certainly have to go without it. Under such circumstances, it is hard to argue that the insurance plan is not practicing medicine but only benignly "administering benefits."

The debate over whether UM saves money is over; it clearly does. Even the prepaid medical groups in California, who have full control over their own use of services and do not face external UM, have found preauthorization and related UM approaches to be a necessary and valuable discipline (Kerr, 1997). In other words, when physicians themselves are at financial risk, they may come to see real value in techniques they once vehemently opposed.

The important controversy surrounding UM focuses on whether it is being applied too vigorously and thus compromising the quality of patient care. At the very least, the denial of payment for hospital services through utilization review denials has generated a public backlash. Witness, for example, the criticism of so-called drive-through deliveries, where women are generally discharged within twenty-four hours after routine childbirth.

Controversies like these have raised the question of who actually is practicing medicine: physicians or the managed care organizations and other payers that have the authority to make medical-necessity decisions. But the competing positions tend to be described in black-and-white terms; the truth is of a grayer shade. When applied improperly, UM can unwisely override the considered judgment of skilled professionals, replacing it with the authority of sometimes inadequately trained individuals and inflexible or flawed utilization review guidelines.

Alternatively, UM can be an effective tool in promoting lower cost and even higher quality. Even the best and most well-intentioned of physicians can make mistakes or be less than fully up-to-speed. Certainly, UM can be abused, but the frequency and extent of that abuse may be less than some would have us believe.

Gatekeepers

Few concepts have become more synonymous with managed care or more symbolic of what it means than the "gatekeeper." Most managed care organizations see gatekeepers as essential to coordinating care in a complex medical world, emphasizing prevention and primary care and making sure that patients see high-cost specialists only when they really need to. To many consumers, however, the gatekeeper is a symbol of managed care's excessive drive to deny access to specialists that once was unlimited. Each view can be both right and wrong.

Gatekeepers, more neutrally called "case managers," represent a specialized form of preauthorization. In place of requiring prior approval for services from a member of the managed care organizations staff, gatekeeper systems require health plan members to select a single physician or group practice on whom they rely to provide or arrange all their medical services. Although gatekeeper systems are commonly associated with HMOs, they actually are not unique to the United States. A number of countries including Great Britain, the Netherlands and Sweden, impose this same requirement on citizens as part of their national health systems.

Even in America it used to be commonplace for patients to develop long-term relationships with a general practitioner who cared for the whole family. When the patient had an unusual problem, this physician arranged for consultation by a specialist. But as specialists became more ubiquitous, patients armed with fee-for-service insurance began to go directly to ophthalmologists, cardiologists, orthopedists, and others, thereby reducing the significance of a relationship with a primary care provider. When managed care began employing the gatekeeper approach to in effect reinstate elements of the old system, it was a recipe for resentment.

In its ideal form, the gatekeeper's role is to coordinate all care for a patient, consulting with or referring to specialized expertise when appropriate. The theory is that by requiring one physician to act as official coordinator of care, relevant clinical information will not be overlooked and costly and sometimes harmful duplication of effort, as well as unnecessary tests and procedures, will be reduced. One common mishap in the fee-for-service system, for example, occurs when two noncommunicating physicians each prescribe medications that are incompatible when taken together. Furthermore, generalist physicians sometimes complain that specialists have become so technology-oriented that they forget they are caring for real people and not just "organ systems." For many reasons then, including the value of a "human" factor, having a designated case manager can be important to a high-quality managed care organization.

Of course, as with all of the techniques used by managed care, there is another side to this argument. Medical specialization took off in part because of the increasing complexity of medicine itself. Many specialists wonder how generalists can possibly stay current enough to oversee complex cases that demand up-to-date and specialized expertise. Many express skepticism, even disdain, for generalists' capacity to deal with such circumstances. Why, they may ask, should a generalist be overseeing care for a patient with heart disease, when a number of studies have shown that cardiologists are more skilled than general physicians in carrying out clinical activities that produce better outcomes for patients with common forms of heart disease (Ayanian and others, 1994; Jollis and others, 1996).

For many clinical problems, this concern is certainly appropriate. In many circumstances, especially those involving chronic illness, the best clinical approach is for a specialist to directly monitor the problem. For example, most primary care physicians are simply not qualified to properly provide ongoing care for a patient with glaucoma or a woman with recurrent breast cysts. In these situations, patients are better off with an ongoing relationship with the specialist, many of whom, in fact, have developed unique interpersonal skills for patients with these particular clinical problems. Good gatekeeper programs should be able to distinguish among clinical problems, encouraging ongoing care from a specialist where necessary.

Unfortunately, to date, gatekeeper approaches have often been cruder than that and have limited direct access to virtually all specialty care, regardless of the circumstances.

Today, managed care plans seem well aware of the pros and cons of gatekeepers and of public skepticism regarding them. Many are revisiting the strategy. Some have even abandoned formal gatekeeper programs. One particular area of controversy has been in the provision of gynecologic services. Many women have objected to the policy that important reproductive health services, including PAP smears, would be performed by primary care physicians and not by gynecologists. In response, many HMOs have adopted a policy that an annual visit to a gynecologist is allowed without a referral from a gatekeeper. A few states have actually made this policy an HMO requirement. With this precedent in place, specialists of all kinds are arguing for special status that would allow patients to bypass gatekeepers and go directly to their care.

New ways of paying for health care

As we have discussed, the single most glaring flaw in the old system was the blank check it gave to physicians and patients, that made it easy to adopt an attitude of "when in doubt, do it." HMOs and other managed care plans try to reverse those incentives. They try to make participating physicians function within a budget. In this way, they send physicians a very different signal: do what is needed—hopefully not less than that—but not more than what is necessary for the patient's well-being. Prepayment thus highlights the values of administrative and clinical efficiency. Savings are profits.

In the best of worlds, prepayment has attributes associated not just with lower cost but with higher quality. It offers reasons to eliminate the fragmentation of care that is inherent in traditional insurance systems. For example, in a fragmented cottage industry in which doctors receive a separate fee for each discrete service they provide, it is difficult to establish a new, more coordinated approach to asthma care, even if it has been proven to produce better results. Doctors are paid for visits, pharmacists for filling prescriptions, and hospitals for emergency room services. But no one gets paid anything for a phone consultation that reduces the need for a visit to a specialist or hospitalization. Nor is there reimbursement for educating a family about how to use pulmonary tests at home or how to properly administer a medication inhaler that might spare the patient an emergency room visit. And no one receives financial compensation for designing the new, integrated approach to care in the first place, or for developing affordable educational programs and then translating them into language that patients can understand (Berwick, 1996). In short, a payment system that reimburses individual professionals for providing defined services freezes innovation, undervalues preventive care, and reinforces the system's orientation to caring only for the sick. Prepayment can address these failings.

The concept of prepayment for a defined population of people also supports prevention, integration, and care innovation because it permits resources to be moved within the system and thus make the best use of the money available. Budgetary savings on hospital care can be applied to home care programs that help people stay out of the hospital or recover after a hospital visit. Group practices can hire nurse practitioners to spend part of their time on the phone with patients with chronic illnesses, making sure they are taking their medicine correctly. Programs can hire nutritionists to assist diabetics in losing weight and maintaining their blood sugar at desired levels, thus helping to head off complications that are both dangerous and expensive. In all these ways, prepayment promotes getting the most care for the fewest dollars.

Going All the Way: Capitation

The most ambitious financial incentive system entails a specific type of prepayment called "capitation" that can only be used by HMOs. A physician or a medical group is paid a fixed amount of money—adjusted for the age and gender of the patient—for each member of the plan for whom they are responsible. This "per member per month" (PMPM) amount does not get supplemented, regardless of the actual services provided. Whether a given patient is never seen or is seen fifteen times a year and receives an elaborate battery of tests and procedures, the PMPM payment is the same.

For obvious reasons, capitation provides physicians considerable incentive to hold down costs. Just as HMOs are at risk when purchasers pay them a fixed fee, here the physicians are at risk. If they cannot hold down costs, they risk losing money. Alternatively, if they can contain costs and practice responsible medicine, they will profit over the long run.

The concept is simple enough, but variations on the capitation theme are almost limitless. Capitation payments may be made to individual physicians, primary care groups, specialty groups, multispecialty groups, or even fully integrated delivery systems that cover all care, including hospital care. Capitation payments can also vary by the number of services covered, from primary care only to all medical services. And they may be adjusted and varied with "bonuses" or "withholds" based on an almost unlimited variety of factors, such as numbers of referrals to specialists or hospitals or ratings on patient satisfaction surveys. The limitless variety of capitation approaches led one consulting firm to calculate, in jest, that there are over 476,000 ways of paying physicians (Governance Committee, 1993).

Whatever the details, capitation has proven as controversial as any element in managed care. To supporters, capitating physicians, like prepayment to an HMO, encourages physicians to be more efficient, to make the best use of all providers—from nurses to the most skilled and experienced subspecialists—and to develop innovative approaches for both individuals and populations that might not be possible under traditional payment mechanisms. In addition, capitation supports a heightened interest in prevention and educational outreach to all plan enrollees, including even the 30 percent who do not see a physician in any given year. For many clinical conditions, including asthma and diabetes, anticipating and heading off a complication may produce care that is both less expensive and of a higher quality than waiting to treat the complication once it has developed.

Use of Selected Measures to Modify Primary Care Physician's Compensation, by Plan Type, 1994
(Percentage of Responding Plans)

Measure to Modify Compensation	All Plans	Group/ Staff HMOs	Network/ IPA HMOs	PPOs
Consumer surveys	36	37	55	3
Quality measures	46	54	64	7
Patient complaints and grievances	49	57	61	21
Enrollee turnover rates	21	11	36	3
Provider productivity	24	43	26	3
Utilization or cost measures	107	28	50	29

Source: Physician Payment Review Commission, 1995.

Finally, capitation can encourage physicians to create integrated or organized systems of care, with untold potential to promote quality and return clinical decision making to physicians. A fully integrated provider organization capable of accepting responsibility for managing both care and costs—that is, accepting "full risk"—is in the best position to follow through on the logic of managed care. It may also be the only organization capable of reorganizing the delivery of care. And most important, from the physicians' point of view, the fully integrated, at-risk provider organization—not the insurer—actually controls the delivery of care. Those physicians who recognize this possibility often see capitation as a means, rather than as a threat, to physician autonomy and control over medical care.

On the other hand, risk taking is risky. It is all too easy to see how capitation payments can work in ways that are not quite so positive from the patient's point of view. Capitated payments may, for example, be insufficient to properly care for assigned patients. A physician or medical group worried about losing patients may agree to a PMPM rate that is simply too low. To try to get by, they may cut corners of care—on tests, procedures, or referrals—thereby threatening the health of patients. Physicians may also find that due to the luck of the draw or their excellent reputations, a particular capitated doctor or group may attract and care for a group of patients who are much sicker patients than average, yet the capitation rates are not adjusted to take into account the patients' illness burden faced by the physicians, in which case the physician may have to choose between providing the care patients need and maintaining his or her own income.

For the consumer, the virtues of capitation can seem pretty theoretical and the dangers very real. The supposed value of an integrated delivery system may be no match for the fear that capitation may encourage physicians to place their financial interests before the needs of their patients.

THE TOOLS IN ACTION

In Chapter 3, we presented the results of a study demonstrating the apparent overuse of cardiac catheterization after heart attacks. Catheterization involves threading a narrow tube into the patient's coronary arteries and then injecting dye to determine the extent of blockage by fatty plaques. Although reasonably safe, performance of the procedure, especially in the aftermath of a heart attack, can result in serious complications. Because of these attendant risks, even without any consideration of cost, performance of this procedure should be carried out only where it is likely to provide a benefit to the patient. Yet, Texas cardiologists do it twice as often as do New York cardiologists, while their patients experience higher mortality rates than those in New York (Guadagnoli and others, 1995).

Because of the risks involved and the expense—as much as $5,000—managed care organizations have a natural interest in trying to make certain that the procedure is performed only when necessary. Their various efforts to achieve this goal provide a good case study in the use of managed care tools.

Selective contracting may be the first tool applied. In contracting with specialists, individually or as a group, a plan might use what information is available to seek out physicians who have records of performing the procedure safely and prudently—in this case, more like New York cardiologists than Texans. In addition, as part of the network selection process, the managed care organizations and the cardiologists might agree in advance on how certain common conditions, such as heart attacks, should be handled. Such agreements or the establishment of practice guidelines that the cardiologists follow might reduce the need for the managed care organizations to impose preauthorization requirements each time a physician decides to use the procedure. Instead of requiring such case-by-case evaluations, the MCO can retrospectively profile the performance of each cardiologist against either explicit guidelines or against his or her peers. If one cardiologist performed, say, 30 percent more catheterizations than the group average, his or her cases might be reviewed in more detail to see if there was clinical justification for this deviation. If not, the physician might be monitored and, if the pattern were not changed, be subject to termination from the plan's network.

Tools involving financial incentives may also be brought to bear. While most specialists today are still paid on a fee-for-service basis, increasing numbers, especially those in groups, are paid by capitation. When paid in this fashion, cardiologists have more incentive to conserve resources and thus to reduce the numbers of unnecessary catheterizations. As a result, managed care organizations, again, should feel less need to impose case-by-case procedures aimed at reducing overutilization. Capitation may also encourage physicians to be more wary of the risks associated with the procedure. They will not, after all, be paid more should complications arise.

Managed care organizations are also almost certain to invoke some form of utilization management, although the review process may differ depending on how physicians are paid. If it makes capitated payments, the responsible plan will need to watch out for underutilization. It will need to monitor contracted physicians, watching for those who may be performing the procedure less frequently than others. It will also need to be sensitive to consumer complaints of underservice.

If, on the other hand, physicians are paid per procedure—fee-for-service—the plan will need to watch for overutilization and the utilization review will likely focus on preauthorization. Using a review protocol that describes specific clinical indications for performing cardiac catheterization, a review nurse would determine whether the cardiologist's recommendation to proceed with a catheterization "meets criteria." If it does, the procedure would proceed. If it does not, the nurse typically would ask a physician advisor, often a cardiologist, to review the case and perhaps to discuss it with the requesting cardiologist to gain additional information or to explain the reason for the rejection. Should the reviewing physician reject the request for the procedure, the physician might then appeal the denial to another review level. At this point, most plans would provide appeals reviewed by physicians who had not been involved in reviewing the case, ideally neutral, uninterested physicians. In an unusual situation, the patient might pursue their rights through plan grievance procedures. They could even, if still dissatisfied, take the matter to court.

Practicing physicians, of course, may object to "second guessing" by health plan personnel who are distant to the doctor-patient relationship. Nevertheless, given the elective nature of the procedure—i.e., it does not have to be performed as an emergency—the patient risks involved, its significant cost, and excess utilization of the catheterization procedure by some physicians, a preauthorization process using well-trained personnel at all levels would seem both appropriate and reasonable.

Finally, gatekeepers may also play a role in reducing unnecessary catheterizations. HMOs and even PPOs might rely on gatekeeper programs and financial incentives applied to primary care physicians to moderate the amount of care provided by specialists such as cardiologists. The gatekeeper, a generalist physician, may have to approve the treatment plan recommended by the cardiologist. In this way, the cardiologist would have to provide a clinical justification to another physician whose role is to coordinate the patient's care and who does not benefit financially from the performance of the procedure. The gatekeeper physician may also be relied on to refer patients to cardiologists whose styles and patterns of practice indicate safe and prudent use of the catheterization procedure. As in the case of selective contracting or capitation, when a gatekeeper serves this role, the need for more intrusive utilization review procedures may be reduced.

As we will discuss further in Chapter 5, health plans might supplement these basic tools—selective contracting, financial incentives, utilization review, and gatekeepers—with other managed care approaches. For example, participating cardiologists might themselves establish practice guidelines that balance considerations of quality and cost. Such guidelines, even if voluntary, could encourage cardiologists to modify their clinical performance to comply with reasonable standards of care. Additionally, a plan might pay for doctors to attend educational courses on management of heart attack patients or might provide data to them on how their utilization compares to their peers'. They might also install computerized medical information search capabilities so that physicians can have on-line information that provides them with results of the most recently published studies relevant to the decision on when to perform catheterization on patients after heart attacks.

Unfortunately, only those HMOs that tend to have exclusive relationships with a group of physicians are likely to engage in these kinds of collaborative educational programs that increase the inherent capabilities of physicians to practice competently and cost-effectively. In the larger and looser networks that characterize IPA-model HMOs and PPOs, building collaborative relationships has proven much more difficult. In these less integrated managed care models, plans tend to rely on financial incentives or the more intrusive tool of preauthorization to control utilization. As a result, these plans may be able to reduce the numbers of unnecessary procedures, but have less capacity to improve the overall quality of care delivered.

CONCLUSION

The tools of managed care—how they are used and what they represent—stand at the center of much of today's controversy over managed care. They are also the focus of an ongoing struggle between providers and health plans. The ability to selectively contract fundamentally changes the power relationship between plans and providers. Preauthorization and gatekeeper programs impose structure on physician decision making and generate a shift of emphasis from specialty to primary care. Capitation and other incentive-payment systems attempt to influence physicians to adopt a more prudent attitude toward the use of expensive technologies and procedures.

As suggested at the outset of this chapter, all of the tools of managed care can be used both to control costs and to improve quality. But to date at least, they have been employed more frequently and with greater effect in the cause of controlling costs than in the search for improving quality. Partly for this reason they have generated great skepticism among consumers, who tend to view the new tools as means by which others make or save money, while their access to services is restricted.

We will explore the possible causes of this trend later in this text. For now, we turn to a second generation of managed care tools, those dedicated more to quality improvement. Given the ongoing emphasis on the use of tools to lower cost, it should not be surprising that these newer tools generally exist more on the drawing board than on the playing field. Still, they are important to understanding the logic and potential of managed care.

5
The
Cutting Edge
of Quality
Improvement

Good
Vibrations

In spite of their potential to improve quality, the core tools of managed care may always have been primarily directed at controlling costs. But as managed care has matured, another set of tools has emerged that would appear to be more dedicated to quality improvement, and especially to improvements in care for those with more complicated medical conditions.

When compared to the tools described in Chapter 4, these second-generation approaches depend more heavily on positive collaboration and integration amongst teams of practitioners and between practitioners and other elements of a managed care organization. In fact, it is largely because of the need for collaboration between the plan and its providers that most managed care organizations have, as yet, been unable to effectively implement them. With the notable exception of the traditional group practice and staff model HMOs, most managed care organizations have not achieved the levels of teamwork and coordination that these approaches require. Indeed, most managed care organizations are still plagued by considerable tension between providers and plans. Moreover, current trends are leading toward less, not more, coordination and integration in managed care arrangements.

Still, these newer and more demanding tools hold considerable potential for quality improvement that is almost certainly unattainable by physicians practicing independently or as part of fragmented systems of care. Thus, they offer an appealing view of the potential of managed care systems to reengineer health care delivery. We outline them here with that potential in mind—reality is far behind—drawing examples from those plans and providers who have been most effective in developing and utilizing these strategies.

QUALITY IMPROVEMENT PROGRAMS AND PRACTICE GUIDELINES

Internal quality improvement programs are generally directed by a formal, designated quality assurance committee and can encompass more than a dozen separate activities. These activities may include focused studies of identified clinical problem areas; identification of "centers of excellence" for high-risk and high-technology services; rigorous credentialing of affiliated practitioners; preventive medicine audits; provider peer review; and member satisfaction surveys. In terms of scope, quality improvement programs can range from the investigation of specific patient grievances to the kinds of sophisticated "continuous quality improvement" approaches that have been used successfully in other industries.

One example of such activities undertaken by many quality assurance committees is the development and implementation of clinical practice guidelines, or systematically developed recommended practice statements created to assist practitioners in making decisions about appropriate care for specific clinical conditions (Siren and Laffel, 1996). Practice guidelines attempt to introduce a level of agreement on how to diagnose and treat common medical problems such as chronic back pain or hypertension, so as to increase the chances for consistent treatment and positive outcomes.

This, of course, can mean the reduction of clinically unwarranted procedures or treatments, such as unnecessary cardiac catheterizations after heart attacks. But clinical guidelines can also serve to protect against underservice, for example, by recommending that heart attack patients be placed on beta blockers, which, as discussed earlier, can decrease the risk of a subsequent heart attack.

A few years ago, an expert panel convened under the auspices of the federal Agency for Health Care Policy and Research (AHCPR) issued a practice guideline on the treatment of acute low back pain, a problem that is treated by many different types of practitioners, including primary care physicians, orthopedists, osteopaths, chiropractors, and physical therapists. Given the array of treatments, a purpose of the back-pain guideline was to clarify what the role of each of the approaches was, based on a review of available scientific evidence and the opinions of experts from the various professions that treat back pain.

The resulting AHCPR guideline became highly controversial because it minimized the role of surgery. In contrast to actual practice in some parts of the country, the guideline reserved major surgery for unusual circumstances and instead recommended other treatment modalities, including medication, physical therapy, chiropractic manipulations, and other noninvasive approaches. Thus, billions of dollars in medical costs could be saved by following these guidelines, at no harm to patient welfare. In response, an organized group of back surgeons denounced the guideline and sought to have AHCPR defunded (Lewis, 1995).

Vulnerable to criticism because it is a federal agency, AHCPR no longer convenes experts to issue practice guidelines to help educate practitioners. Nevertheless, many organizations outside of government, including medical specialty societies and managed care organizations, continue to develop or adapt guidelines because of the evident need to standardize practice. Managed care organizations either develop their own or adapt guidelines developed elsewhere for their own use.

Ideally, practice guidelines should be based on the best available knowledge, usually gathered in a review of data found in scientific journals. They serve as evidence-based approaches of proper care for specific clinical problems. Importantly, guidelines are generally used in an advisory capacity only; as the term implies, guidelines are not a set of mandated rules. Still, some managed care organizations may attempt to monitor compliance with guidelines with the goal of identifying and even sanctioning physicians who without clinical justification consistently deviate from the recommended approach.

Possibly because of their advisory nature and the general lack of effective oversight of physicians' practice, it does not appear that practice guidelines have resulted in significant changes in clinical practice, at least as measured by the persistence of large variations in physician practice patterns (Kosecoff and others, 1987; Lomas and others, 1989). Moreover, to accommodate uncertain scientific data and different opinions, many practice guidelines have been written so generally that they can accommodate almost any practice approach, thereby undercutting their purpose.

Finally, utilization of guidelines is complicated by the reality that there is no guideline gold standard. There are literally thousands of clinical practice guidelines, and even dozens that address the same topic, such as the appropriate management of low back pain or hypertension. The result is that physicians who contract with many managed care organizations—i.e., most physicians—may be expected to follow somewhat different guidelines for the same clinical problem, just as they are expected to comply with multiple utilization review processes.

It should come as no surprise, then, that physicians complain about and resist bureaucratic overload. The paradoxical result can be that even well-intentioned efforts of an managed care organization to achieve the best care for its enrollees encounter resistance from the best intentioned of physicians. Clearly, the problem may not lie with either the managed care organization or the physician, but with the interaction of each with too many of the other.

Quality assurance committees also have responsibility for oversight of the health plan's performance, as measured by external organizations producing "report cards" that permit purchasers and consumers to compare and choose plans. The most prominent report card, called the Healthplan Employer Data and Information Set and known by the unappealing acronym HEDIS, was developed by the National Committee of Quality Assurance (NCQA), the national accrediting body for HMOs and has undergone several iterations. Many, but by no means all, HMOs submit HEDIS data to NCQA, which arrays it on a comparative report card of plans. By reviewing the HEDIS report, purchasers can, for example, compare the rates of childhood immunization, the rates of avoidable asthma hospital admissions, and the percentage of plan members who are satisfied with the plan.

The goal of the process is not simply to provide more information to purchasers, but to encourage plans to undertake, with their participating physicians, quality enhancing programs that will enable them to improve performance. As we will emphasize later, most employers today make minimal if any use of HEDIS or other report cards. Nevertheless, with NCQA accreditation requirements and HEDIS performance measures in place, many HMOs and some PPOs have been pressed to put quality improvement strategies in place, even if only for the reason that markets and purchasers may soon demand them.

DEMAND MANAGEMENT

At least in some quarters, managed care suffers because of its proclivity for using the business term "management" to define activities that attempt to improve health care for patients and populations. (In fact, long before the ascendance of managed care, physicians commonly referred to their activities as "managing patients.") Following this convention, HMOs have adopted the term "demand management" to refer to a number of activities designed to reduce the overall requirement for health services by plan members. Although designed partly to reduce patient demand for services and thereby hold down costs, these programs could also prove highly appealing to patients who can experience reduced dependence on physician care, more control over their own health, and more opportunity to maintain and improve their health status.

For example, nurse advice lines provide members with direct telephone access to informed advice on preventive care and on when to seek medical care for specific problems. When staffed by appropriately trained individuals, such advice lines can reduce the need for office or even emergency room visits, saving money for the plan and inconvenience for the member. As another element of a demand management strategy, health plans commonly provide newsletters to members that feature information on self-care for common problems and reminders on when and how often various preventive measures should be taken.

At a more sophisticated level, some health plans now encourage or even require patients with specific medical problems for which there are alternative treatment options—for example, prostate cancer—to complete a "shared decision-making program." These programs use interactive CD-ROM, videotape, and computer software to engage the patient and family members so that they can become more active and knowledgeable participants in decisions that were once left to the "professionals." The videos present the latest scientific evidence on likely clinical outcomes of alternative treatments and include perspectives from other patients who have faced similar alternatives.

For example, videos on options relating to treatment of symptomatic prostatic enlargement emphasize that, as is often the case with elective surgery, "watchful waiting" is often a reasonable alternative to surgery. The video reviews the specific pros, cons, and potential risks of "watchful waiting" as opposed to surgery. Perhaps, not surprisingly, when shown the video, large numbers of men choose to wait, thereby avoiding the major surgery known as transurethral prostatectomy that was for years the gold standard treatment (Millenson, 1997b).

Managed care does not deserve primary credit for developing these and other approaches to patient participation in health care decision making. Nevertheless, the organizational capacity of managed care plans and an increased emphasis on prevention and self-help can produce an environment that is more conducive to shared decision making than the old professional-dominated environment that tended toward paternalism and lacked the capital to mount demand-management programs. Although the use of demand management is limited today and mostly to reducing costs, expansion of its focus could provide a much-needed reorientation in how clinical decisions are made. And while initially resistant, many physicians will likely recognize the improvement in care that would result from better informed patients.

PROGRAMS FOR THE CATASTROPHICALLY AND CHRONICALLY ILL

One of the major concerns about MCOs generally and HMOs in particular is that they are oriented to the care of relatively healthy persons—for whom even managed care critics acknowledge they do a pretty good job—but tend to skimp on care for those with major illnesses, particularly those with debilitating chronic illnesses. Indeed, the basic tools of managed care, described in Chapter 4, seem designed primarily with a relatively healthy patient population in mind. For example, requiring enrollees to be seen first by a gatekeeper makes sense for patients who may have a number of straightforward medical problems that need care and coordination. However, it may be a more dubious strategy for care of a chronically ill patient in need of ongoing specialty care. Similarly, capitation payments— although they may be calculated on an assumption that some of the patients covered will require the expenditure of a lot of money—may still leave physicians viewing high-cost patients as threats to their ability to turn a reasonable profit. Faced with these doubts, and given the reality that they will inevitably enroll patients with significant chronic health problems even if they try to avoid doing so, some managed care organizations have developed programs designed specifically to improve the care provided to these patients.

One such tool, sometimes employed by traditional insurers as well as HMOs and PPOs, is called "large case management." It refers to focused techniques for identifying and overseeing individual patients with catastrophic or otherwise extraordinarily expensive medical problems.

Patients whose conditions may attract such special attention include those who sustain a spinal cord injury, suffer from severe burns, have active AIDS, or receive bone marrow transplants. Effective care for patients with these and other catastrophic problems typically includes mobilization of various health professionals with diverse skills—physicians, nurses, rehabilitation therapists, psychotherapists, etc.—as well as the active involvement of family members and other community-based support services. The goal is to coordinate the health care and other efforts of all the parties involved so as to anticipate and handle the complicated problems these patients invariably encounter.

The insurance company itself—apart from the medical delivery system—often needs to play a central role in organizing the effort because implementing the best care plan often involves interpreting or adjusting the patient's insurance-benefit package. For example, the patient's insurance may include only limited coverage for durable medical equipment such as a motorized wheelchair or hospital bed. Yet, it may be in both the patient's and the plan's best interests to provide the equipment so that the patient can leave the hospital and go home.

As is the case with all managed care tools, large case management can be used primarily as a mechanism to save money; insurers are less willing to waive benefit exclusions if the resultant care becomes more expensive than it would have been. Nevertheless, where large case management does take place, the enhanced flexibility provided is likely to produce benefits for the patient and family.

DISEASE MANAGEMENT

Still another approach, also involving considerable coordination among health care professionals, has been labeled "disease management." These programs are targeted to patients with those chronic illnesses—e.g., asthma, diabetes, and congestive heart failure—that require more coordinated effort than a fragmented system of independent practitioners can generally produce. The approach emphasizes the value of augmenting physician care, usually provided by a specialist, with efforts of nonphysician practitioners who become expert in caring for patients with the target condition. Just as with large case management, disease management rejects the fee-for-service orientation that medical care is provided only by physicians and only for discrete encounters with the health care system. A fee-for-service orientation may be appropriate for treatable and resolvable acute clinical problems such as a broken limb or a bout of influenza or appendicitis. But for chronic conditions, in which symptoms may wax and wane but never disappear, an emphasis on prevention, on coordination of caregivers, and on patient and family involvement in decision making can offer obvious advantages.

Accordingly, disease management programs are compatible with prepayment and capitation, but not with fee-for-service payment strategies. For example, numerous studies have concluded that periodic phone calls to patients with congestive heart failure, probing how they are doing and whether they are taking their medication in the right amounts and at the right times, can decrease complication rates, hospitalizations, and doctor visits (Rich and others, 1995). Yet, traditional fee-for-service programs do not reimburse physician practices for telephone calls and, consequently, telephone monitoring of how patients are doing is underutilized in fee-for-service practice. In contrast, prepayment permits and encourages an organization to make best use of personnel—physician and nonphysician—without regard to whether a discrete service will be reimbursed.

In his recent and compelling book *Demanding Medical Excellence*, author Michael Millenson (1997b) chronicles a particular example of how a disease management program focused on asthma can dramatically improve care and patient well-being. The example comes from the Harvard Pilgrim Health Plan, formerly the Harvard Community Health Center, one of the most respected HMOs in the country. (In virtually all of the report cards that compare HMO performance, Harvard Pilgrim is near the top of the pack.)

As documented by Millenson, asthma has become one of the most prevalent chronic diseases of childhood, responsible for more than 10 million school days, some 200,000 hospitalizations of children, and an increasing number of avoidable asthma deaths. In fact, in the midst of major improvements in health care technology and available medications, the death rate from asthma has actually doubled since 1980. The Harvard health plan's disease management program for asthma care was aimed at addressing this serious health problem by easing the burden of illness for the patients under its care (Millenson, 1997b).

The program first used its comprehensive database of drug prescriptions, hospital admissions, and emergency room visits to identify patients with asthma. By reviewing the medical records of the individuals who had sought care in its system, the health plan identified more than 3,000 asthmatic adults and children and their doctors in its Boston-area health centers. In essence, Harvard did what rarely occurs in fee-for-service medicine or even in most managed care organizations: it systematically identified patients at risk for certain untoward health events in order to intervene before these events occurred.

The plan next educated all of its physicians on the modern treatment of asthma, about which many conscientious physicians simply are unaware. They then borrowed from the recommended guidelines of a panel of asthma experts organized by the National Institutes of Health and developed a Harvard-specific practice guideline for general application across the health plan. For example, the guideline taught physicians that asthma requires the routine use of inhaled corticosteroids, a recommendation that was new to some physicians. The program also educated doctors and nurses on how to teach patients to properly self-administer an inhaler, and then instructed children and their parents in using peak-flow meters, which permit patient self-evaluation of the force of their breathing at home. Patients or their parents could then routinely monitor their condition and modify prescribed medications in order to reduce flare-ups of asthma and, in particular, serious exacerbations that in the absence of self-administration of appropriate medication might quickly develop into life-threatening attacks.

Through these and other straightforward but previously neglected disease management approaches, the Harvard health plan's program was able to reduce hospital admissions for asthma by 86 percent and emergency room visits by 79 percent in the initial pilot study. In short, the program produced benefits in lower costs and in improved quality of life for patients and their families.

So far, disease management programs have focused on chronic medical problems—e.g., asthma, congestive heart failure, and some forms of diabetes—for which payoff in improved health and reduced costs can be achieved in a short time. Yet, other chronic diseases should be amenable to this multidisciplinary approach as well. With reforms that we will recommend in Chapter 10—in particular, risk adjustment of premiums to take into account the burden of illness of patients who join plans—managed care organizations may expand disease management beyond its current use. And, to play a broken record, organizations that engage a limited number of physicians in a collaborative environment can use the disease management approach much more effectively than those that affiliate with virtually all of the providers in the community.

SPECIALTY BENEFIT CARVE-OUTS

HMO members have learned, sometimes to their surprise, that care for a particular set of benefits is actually under the direction of a separate organization with which their HMO has contracted. In particular, it is very common for mental health and substance abuse services to be "carved out" from the medical benefits provided by the HMO's own network of providers. In this example, the HMO negotiates a capitated monthly payment with a behavioral health company that maintains its own provider network and performs other functions, including utilization management, that otherwise would be performed by the HMO itself.

The theory underlying benefit carve-outs is similar to that underlying disease management, that the clinical problems involved are so unique that they are most appropriately managed by specialists in that particular field. However, in contrast to the disease management approach in which the managed care organization plays an active role, carve-outs involve turning over the management of the care to a separate organization.

The organization accountable for the carved-out services may, like most managed care organizations, be a loose network of providers and other professionals who rarely interact with each other or a tightly integrated organization in which the various types of professionals routinely work together. In the loose network, the carve-out company may still be able to focus attention on cost control and reduced utilization of services. However, it will have great difficulty engaging providers in the kinds of coordinated effort required for quality improvement in complex cases.

By contrast, when the carved-out services are provided by an organization dedicated to comprehensive care to patients suffering a particular health problem, the care provided may be very different. For example, a comprehensive program dedicated to oncology will strive to coordinate the services of physician oncologists with the efforts of other medical specialists, home care nurses, nutritionists, counselors, and other skilled personnel. Theoretically at least, such a capability can lead to both higher quality and more affordable services (Herzlinger, 1997).

Carve-out programs are controversial, to be sure, because in some circumstances they may actually undermine rather than improve coordination of care. That is because some patients, particularly seniors in the Medicare population, may well have multiple health problems that need coordination and continuity that might not be supported with a series of carve-out programs. Also, directing all patients with a discrete health problem such as cancer or depression to a specialized organization may be resisted by many patients who continue to want to see their own physicians or be admitted to their own community hospital. For these and other reasons, disease management and benefit carve-outs are works in progress. Their precise role in improving the quality of care for patients with chronic health problems will evolve as managed care matures.

THE LOGIC OF MANAGED CARE MEETS REALITY

The disease management program for asthma at Harvard Pilgrim Health Plan costs more than $1 million annually. It entails extensive levels of coordination and information sharing that, in turn, require sophisticated information systems. It requires systemwide agreement on clinical guidelines and a sizable organizational investment in ongoing physician education. Promotion of such a strategy may even require that significant numbers of professionals—physicians and nonphysicians— have a common organizational home and a common economic bottom line.

The same can be said about other managed care tools, especially the second generation of managed care approaches outlined in this chapter. They are likely to work most effectively when health care professionals are functioning in a collaborative, joint enterprise. In a word, efforts like this require "organization." They cannot be implemented in the fragmented world of independent practitioners and fee-for-service medicine.

Efforts like the Harvard Pilgrim asthma program also provide a glimpse into how, when properly constituted, managed care organizations can produce clear benefits for their enrollees by both controlling costs and improving quality. This is the logic and potential of managed care.

But today's reality rarely approaches that logic or potential. If anything, today's dominant market trends actually moving in the direction of less coordination and integration in managed care plans. The plans growing fastest are those offering the most choice; those offering the most in integration, the traditional group practice models, are generally growing slowly, if at all. Moreover, rather than associating with one or a few plans, physicians today are likely to have contracts with literally dozens of managed care or self-insured health benefits plans. Each plan may have its own contracting procedures, its own unique preauthorization requirements and protocols, its own variations on paying physicians, and its own concept of a gatekeeper.

In such an environment, even the best intentioned of managed care organizations will be hard-pressed to effectively apply the tools of the trade and physicians, for their part, will be more likely to view those tools as onerous, intrusive, and bureaucratic. Health plan-developed practice guidelines will be, at best, a nuisance to physicians who must live with guidelines provided by a dozen or more competing plans. Educational efforts to help physicians get up-to-speed or to assist them in installing computer systems to improve care management will, in effect, be offering assistance to competing companies who contract with the same physicians. The capacity to implement a disease management-type program will remain undeveloped.

At best, the tools will still be capable of asserting some control on costs, although if the trend to large, undifferentiated networks of providers continues, even that success could be jeopardized. But, in the absence of more integrated structures, the tools of managed care will have little capacity to improve quality.

As we will endeavor to explain later in the text, the causes of this failure and of the trends underlying it cannot be laid at any one doorstep. After years of double-digit inflation in premiums, the employer purchaser has demanded lower premiums and has been far less concerned about improving quality. Cost savings are easily measured, but quality, unfortunately, still remains largely in the eye of the beholder. With a few notable exceptions, purchasers have not demanded better quality for their money.

Plans have responded by competing aggressively on price but not on quality. They have been able to reduce costs by wringing out the excesses and inefficiencies of the old system and by using their growing market power to demand that providers do as much for less. But they have not yet seen a compelling need to reengineer the delivery of health care. Even worse, many HMOs and other managed care plans actively resist efforts by hospitals and physicians to forge integrated delivery systems focused around group practice principles that could be capable of managing financial risk. After all, those systems might soon become competitors of insurers and raise questions about the "value" added by the insurer.

Physicians, for their part, while more likely to join group practices in recent years, have done so primarily for defensive reasons—to fight managed care, not to collaborate with or lead it. Many continue to resist the multidisciplinary team concept and view even reasonable attempts to oversee their performance as unconscionable threats to their autonomy and authority.

Finally, the American consumer/patient, fearful that managed care means poor-quality care, may take refuge in a demand for choice of physician. Choice has become the surrogate for quality, but it actually may do more to undermine than promote it. As employers and plans respond to consumer demands for choice, the drive to integration and coordination recedes into a marketplace with every doctor participating in every plan.

For all these reasons, the integration and coordination that is so critical to quality improvement seems to hold limited appeal to those who need to sign on—purchasers, plans, physicians, and patients. Indeed, many appear to view these critical components of quality improvement as more threat than asset. Thus, as managed care has succeeded in holding down costs, it has paid a price in increasing concern about the quality of care provided. One result has been a counterattack or backlash that may have the capacity to both improve and undermine the search for quality in managed care.

6
The Managed Care Backlash | *Stop in the Name of Love*

Robert Raible produces an Internet web page entitled "Fight Managed Care" (www.his.com\~pico\usa.htm). It features regularly updated summaries of managed care "horror stories" from newspapers around the country, along with information about pending managed care legislation and how to support or fight it. It also reprints polls—at least those featuring growing public concerns with managed care.

But the "horror story" summaries are the focal point. (You get to them by clicking on the image of Picasso's "Guernica," a terrifying view of the bombing of that town by Franco's forces in the Spanish Civil War.) The summaries make for chilling reading. Each suggests that some managed care organization, presumably driven by bottom-line considerations, lack of concern for patients' well-being, or just gross incompetence, failed to offer necessary or appropriate care, with disastrous results.

As of late 1997 Raible's list ran to over 175 stories and seems to climb almost daily. The headlines are often meant to shock: "Ex-New Yorker Is Told: Get Castrated So We Can $ave (*NY Post*, 9/18/96); "Is Your Doctor Looking Out for You? Or Your Insurer?" (*Philadelphia Inquirer*, 3/24/96); "Assembly Line Medicine?" (*Los Angeles Times*, 8/27/95); "Teacher Battles Cancer and Bureaucracy" (*Syracuse Post-Standard*, 1/22/96); "Woman 'Punished' for Having Chronic Disease" (*Tucson Citizen*, 1/9/96).

Raible works for an association of home health care agencies. Today many of these home care providers are concerned about getting "locked out" of managed care plans. The web page, which is his personal effort (not the organization's), emerged after he had volunteered to compile a series of anecdotes about managed care mishaps. The Internet proved to be fertile ground. He reports that the site has received over 15,000 "hits" and that of the hundreds of e-mail messages he has received about the page, only three have been critical. The horror stories, he admits, can be a bit "strident," but they do capture attention. They also raise important issues at the core of this chapter (Raible, 1997).

The web page and the materials it provides are but one indicator of the ascendant/defendant status of managed care today. The body of concerns they outline about choice, quality, access, profit seeking, and consumer protection in managed care comprises a backlash with few historical precedents.

To be fair, much of the media coverage of managed care is nonsensational and balanced. Even many of the stories with sensationalist headlines turn out to have two sides, both usually credible. But, clearly, whether one- or two-sided, these stories are tapping into, and perhaps fueling, a broad public concern.

That concern, and the backlash that springs from it, can also be seen in public opinion polls. While most polls reveal generally high levels (75 percent or higher) of consumer satisfaction with managed care, they also suggest a number of serious concerns. In August 1997, a Harris and Associates Poll found that 54 percent of Americans believed the trend to managed care is harmful for them, an increase from 43 percent just one year earlier (Kilborn, September 1997). The same poll found the public split, 44 percent to 44 percent, on the question of whether the trend to managed care was a good thing for society in general. But the 44 percent that said it was *not* good for society represented a striking increase from just 28 percent two years earlier. A Kaiser Family Foundation survey in late 1996 found that 51 percent of those questioned believed that government needs to "protect consumers from being treated unfairly" in managed care plans (Hilzenrath, July 1997). And in an early 1997 Harris and Associates Poll, 38 percent of respondents said they believed that managed care companies such as HMOs "generally do a bad job of serving their customers" (Hilzenrath, July 1997). The trend, says Harris Poll Executive Vice-President Robert Leitman, is "definitely . . . toward accelerating levels of dissatisfaction.'"

Even more disturbing evidence came in a late 1997 California poll. It revealed reasonably high levels of consumer satisfaction with managed care, but also showed that a sizable number of respondents reported having had a significant problem with their health insurance. Over 12 percent said they had experienced a problem involving pain and suffering that lasted longer than it should have; 9 percent reported a problem that led to the worsening of their health; and 2 percent claimed that their difficulty with their health plan had led to permanent disability ("Public Perceptions," 1997). Based on poll responses, researchers projected that 1.4 million Californians had experienced a "problem" with their insurance and that they associated it with poorer health ("Public Perceptions," 1997).

Physicians have also stepped up, or at least changed, their critique of managed care. Until recently, that criticism tended to come across as self-serving complaints about the reduction in physician income, autonomy, and authority. Now physicians and their organizations are more likely to focus their critiques on how managed care may harm patient care. Their focus on "gag" clauses, on threats to quality posed by capitation, and on patients' need for greater access to specialty care may still carry an element of self-interest, but it has also led to successful alliances with consumer groups and perhaps to a deeper understanding of where managed care can go wrong.

As patients, polls, press, and providers voice concern, it should surprise no one that the political process is close behind. By 1995, Congress and the state legislatures were flooded with proconsumer or anti-managed care legislation. These proposals represent what we might call the "operational" side of the backlash—where concerns turn into action.

In the last half of 1995 and 1996, nine states passed laws relating to "access problems" with emergency care; 18 states approved legislation guaranteeing consumers direct access to obstetricians and gynecologists (as opposed to going through a gate-keeper); 25 states set length-of-stay standards for new mothers; 15 states prohibited "gag" clauses; nine states mandated additional "due process" protections for physicians being dropped from networks; 13 states strengthened requirements that HMOs provide information to prospective enrollees. (*HMO Consumers at Risk*, 1996). And in 1997 and 1998 hundreds of bills were drafted relating to, among other things, access to specialists, limits on the amount of financial risk that could be passed to physicians, quality assurance requirements, disclosure of financial incentives imposed on physicians, and rights of consumers when faced with denials of care.

At the federal government level, Congress in 1996 enacted legislation to enhance group and individual rights in the small group marketplace. The law, among other things, intended to ease the ability to individuals and groups to move from one insurance plan to another, to restrict the imposition of "pre-existing conditions," and to limit the ability of insurers to charge more to those in poor health. In early 1998, a special commission on quality appointed by President Clinton issued a call for enhanced consumer protection in managed care, including several of the kinds of measures states have been considering. (A similar set of proposals came from a special California commission).

In this chapter and Chapter 7, we will assess the origins of and the concerns embodied in the backlash against managed care. We will look at how accurately the concerns expressed in the backlash reflect the real state of managed care. To what extent does managed care deserve the anger, resentment, and fear that it so commonly inspires? To what extent is it just bearing the brunt of unspoken decisions—made by government, employers, and even society at large—that the old system was broken and that somehow, someone must impose controls on health care spending? Only after we have tried to define what is real and what is not, will we be able to evaluate the solutions, big and small, that have been proposed for managed care's shortcomings.

DISSECTING THE HORROR STORY

Bob Herbert of the *New York Times* often uses his op-ed column to launch attacks on managed care and HMOs in particular. On July 4, 1997, his column titled "A Chance to Survive" detailed the case of a twenty-nine-year-old man with a malignant melanoma that had spread to his brain and lungs—a terminal condition (Herbert, 1997). The patient's oncologist recommended nonstandard, heroic treatment that, in his experience, had prolonged the life of a few other patients.

The HMO, Herbert reports, rejected the proposed treatment as "experimental." The oncologist was outraged. The proposed treatment was not, in his opinion, experimental, and he said he had published data to prove it, although the insurance company had sought opinions of three doctors, each of whom, apparently, had thought the treatment to be experimental. The subsequent indictment, clearly supported by Herbert, has become standard fare. In the words of the oncologist, "This is what we have come to expect. Insurance companies are not in the business of curing people, they are in the business of making money. They will use any excuse to deny payment of what they perceive as more expensive therapy."

It is a sad story, and a classic HMO bashing tale. But does it really represent a fair indictment of managed care? Herbert suggests that the patient and physician know best and that the insurer should not overrule their judgment, no matter what the cost or clinical evidence. But given the cost consequences, we do not find that position very compelling. To argue that a patient in these circumstances should be entitled to a formal review process before an independent panel—as we will recommend later—is one thing. To suggest that the patient's physician is, by definition, correct and should be given a blank check is another.

Moreover, the story—like so many horror story indictments about managed care—is not really about managed care or HMOs; it is about health insurance of any kind. (Indeed, it is not at all clear that the insurance company in Herbert's story was a managed care organization.) Insurers all make more when they pay out less. In this case, even had the patient had a traditional insurance plan, there is every reason to believe that the insurer would have balked at paying. They do it all the time. In fact, some traditional insurance plans balk even more than HMOs. HMOs, at least, have some means of controlling costs; traditional insurers do not. Thus, a case like this one would cost a traditional insurance plan much more than it would cost an HMO. As a result, they may have more reason to deny coverage and refuse payment.

This failure to assess trade-offs reflects an oversimplification that often mars the media's indictment of managed care. For example, in what was generally a carefully researched and well-written series of anecdotes about the failings of managed care entitled *Health against Wealth: HMOs and the Breakdown of Medical Trust*, author George Anders studied the decision of the Health Insurance Plan (HIP) of Greater New York to shift its heart surgery patients from New York Hospital to North Shore Hospital. New York Hospital, Anders informs us, had one of the best heart surgery programs in the state, as measured by post-surgery mortality rates. North Shore had only an "adequate" program, ranking fourteenth out of thirty-one hospitals performing open-heart surgery. HIP, he argues, made the shift simply to reduce the costs of heart surgery. "The only losers," he writes dramatically, "were HIP members with heart disease" (Anders, 1996).

It sounds alarming, and it might be. But Anders does not tell us the magnitude of the savings to HIP for us to assess the reasonableness of the cost-quality trade-off HIP made. Rather, he implies—as do so many others—that no such trade-off is legitimate, that any decision to save money, no matter how much, that in any way reduces quality, no matter how little, is wrong. In fact, the difference in outcomes between the two hospitals, defined in terms of mortality rates that are adjusted for the risk level of the patients served, was less than 1 percent. HIP could further justify its switch if it had used the savings to inaugurate an education program for heart disease patients that might save far more lives than directing its heart surgery patients to New York Hospital.

Anders concludes, "Even at North Shore there was little belief that HIP's choice of this hospital was made for clinical reasons alone" (Anders, 1996). Of course it wasn't. And it shouldn't have been. Quality counts. But so, too, must cost.

Without a doubt, many journalists have risen above the horror story and produced thorough and balanced accounts of managed care. Some of these have detailed real abuses. Such stories reveal, among other things, how the tools of managed care can be misused. But far too many stories leave out critical pieces of information, or treat legitimate trade-offs as cave-ins to a "bottom line," or imply that an isolated practice of one company necessarily reflects a systematic flaw in all. They blame managed care, when the problem, as in the Herbert example, is insurance itself. They indict HMOs when the problem is a physician error that has nothing to do with HMO policies, or they attack managed care for denying access to benefits when the "insurer" is actually a self-insured employer who has decided that a certain procedure would not be covered in its plan. Even when they are factually accurate, many tales are mere anecdotes, individual episodes that may or may not be representative of the truth. One can find as many stories about horrible medical outcomes in the old fee-for-service system that might have been prevented had some managed care tool been effectively in place.

If we are going to understand how managed care is doing when it comes to quality of care, we will need better evidence than anecdotes or horror stories usually offer.

CONSUMER CONCERNS: WHO COMES FIRST?

To say that many of the attacks on managed care are shrill is hardly to suggest that there is no legitimate cause for public concern. Even if managed care had achieved much higher levels of public approval and acceptance than it has, there would still be good reason for consumers to be wary and to demand appropriate protection from potentially inappropriate actions. The hard, though perhaps necessary, reality is that managed care introduces incentives and pressures to restrain costs and access that can—especially when inappropriately applied—threaten consumer rights and raise legitimate fears about quality of care. For better or worse, managed care can dramatically alter how consumers access the health care system and what happens when they do. The extent to which the consumer backlash accurately reflects failings in the constructs or practices of

Highest Users Best Customers?	
Managed Care Highest Users	Airline, Utility, Retailer Highest Users
• Highest cost	• Highest revenue
• Biggest loser	• Biggest profit
• Retention not critical (not wanted?)	• Retention critical
• Level of service provided?	• Level of service unlimited

managed care is a more specific question and one to which we now turn.

In virtually all businesses, the best customers are those the business sees the most. These customers generate the most revenue and the most profit. Businesses will bend over backwards to serve them. Airlines give frequent flyers free upgrades and other rewards. Utilities give their highest users the lowest rates. Smart retailers rarely argue when a regular customer wants to return a product, no matter what the reason. Most important of all, they do almost anything to retain their best customers. The costs of retaining a good customer are much lower than those of recruiting a new customer. All this is part of putting the customer, especially the best customer, first.

But in the prepaid, managed care context all this can get reversed. The customer that a managed care organization most wants to retain is the one it rarely sees. Because the costs are paid up front, the healthy nonuser of services will generate the most profit. By contrast, the diabetic, the senior with Parkinson's disease or the child with cystic fibrosis whom physicians will see on a regular basis will generate the highest costs and the biggest losses. They, or their employers, may pay $1,700 a year in premiums. They may receive thousands, perhaps tens of thousands of dollars in treatment. Consequently, rather than giving its highest user the red-carpet treatment, a health plan may have no problem when its highest user walks out the exit door and enrolls somewhere else. When plan ethics are borderline and economic pressures severe, they may even help them find that door.

As we have noted, this is true of traditional health insurance as well as managed care. Traditional insurance, too, was prepaid. But under the old health insurance system, even if insurers were not happy to see the patient, the physician was. Physicians had no reason to do less or cut costs. Their highest users *were* their best customers.

What people find troubling about managed care is that the pressure to lower costs by doing less is extended, even transferred, from the office of a distant insurer to the office of the physician. Physicians in such cases are said to be "at risk" for services for a group of patients. From the patient's point of view, and sometimes from the physician's as well, this difference is a huge change and can lead to very fundamental questions of trust and confidence.

Even when consumers accept that the old system may have encouraged physicians to do more than necessary, concerns are still real. At some point, the easy savings in reductions in procedures and tests will all have been taken. The "low-hanging fruit" will have been picked. Capitation and other payment arrangements that push physicians to go beyond those savings may then begin to impinge on quality. For such reasons, evidence of flat or falling premiums can alarm those concerned about the new system. Heightened levels of competition between increasingly for-profit managed care organizations that put greater pressure on providers may look good to those paying the premiums. But those receiving the care—even if they are paying part of the bills—may take a different view.

When patients hear about managed care "gag" clauses, or about once nonprofit health plans now needing to serve stockholder and Wall Street interests, or about their physician's exclusion from a plan in which they have been enrolled, concerns about loss of the patient-first ethic grow intense. Proposals to mandate disclosure of physician payment rules, to limit the nature of physician payment arrangements, to ban gag clauses, to support physician-led efforts to open up networks or ease referral restrictions, and a number of other legislative fixes are likely to follow.

CHOICE, ACCESS, AND QUALITY

Limits on choice of physician and access to specialists inherent to most managed care plans are also central to consumer concerns. It may be one thing, as in the old fee-for-service system, to be "locked in" to a particular insurance company. It is clearly another to be "locked out" from one's physician of choice. HMO arguments that limiting choice to a defined network will improve coordination of care and thus quality are not selling yet. Even many consumers who accept the value and logic of a more integrated system will not easily accept rules that say they *cannot* go elsewhere should they think it important to do so.

Demands for physician choice might be less intense if consumers had confidence in the quality of care offered by managed care plans. But, for all kinds of reasons, most do not. Consumers tend to associate quality in health care with a physician or hospital, not an insurer or health plan. They may have an image of quality—accurate or not—of certain well-known national systems like Kaiser Permanente or local HMOs like Northern California's Health Plan of the Redwoods. But what do they know about Aetna, Cigna, Humana, Blue Cross, or other plans that used to pay the claims? As we will see in Chapter 8, the science of assessing quality in health plans is still in its infancy. Few Americans have any experience with comparison shopping for health plans, and—unlike shopping for cars or televisions—they have few tools with which to do it.

In the absence of an ability to judge quality, choice becomes a safety valve. Thus, a direct relationship emerges between the two. The greater the concern about quality, the greater the demand for choice. By contrast, when the consumer is told that he *must* go to the Mayo Clinic, concerns about choice may subside. Consumers' demands for physician choice might also be less intense if they had more flexibility to change plans and thus networks and physicians. But most employers, especially small employers, still offer little if any choice of plan (Jensen, 1997).

Ample research, which we will detail later, suggests that managed care's leaner choice of doctors and limits on access to health services have not harmed the quality of care offered to American consumers. But the average patient is not aware of these findings, which often appear only in academic journals. To patients, managed care looks like it is standing between them and the high-quality, easy-access-to-any-physician health care they used to know. Moreover, consumers may be justifiably suspicious of the "satisfaction" surveys frequently cited by the managed care industry. Eighty percent or more of enrollees may be satisfied with their health plan, but since only a small portion of people get seriously ill in any given year, only a handful of those surveyed have had a chance to see their plan really put to the test.

Such concerns explain the rise of the POS opt-out option and the trend to broader physician networks. They also underlie many legislative proposals aimed at guaranteeing choice of physician or access to specialists and laws guaranteeing payment when "prudent" consumers visit the emergency room. On the quality front, concerns lead to proposals, among others, that would require the collection and dissemination of more quality-oriented data, strengthen grievance procedures, allow patients to seek second opinions, and force plans to contract with various centers of excellence.

THE GREED FACTOR

Whereas, early HMOs were exclusively nonprofit, in recent decades the industry has come to be dominated by for-profit corporations. Between 1988 and 1994, membership in for-profit HMOs went up 92 percent, in part because many nonprofit plans converted to for-profit status. Consumers have not fled for-profit plans for nonprofit ones, but the transition to a for-profit-dominated industry has led to serious misgivings about pressures to raise the bottom line by reducing consumer access to care. The nation's biggest health care company, Columbia/

Comment on Wellpoint Conversion

"This will liberate them from their social responsibilities. They can focus on the things that they need to do to make their business grow."

—Wall Street Analyst

HCA, though a hospital/provider organization and not a health plan, has become a lightning rod for public resentment of the corporatization of medicine, and much of that opposition has spilled over into the managed care world. More Americans now believe that nonprofit health care organizations deliver higher quality care than do for-profits (Kilborn, 1997).

The recent frenzy of hospital and plan merger and acquisition activity has only intensified consumer concerns, especially since it is usually smaller, regionally based organizations that are swallowed up by larger, often national organizations. United HealthCare bought MetraHealth; Humana bought Emphesys; Anthem purchased New Jersey Blue Cross; Aetna bought U.S. Healthcare; and two giant California HMO mergers left about 75 percent of all California HMO enrollees in just four plans.

Reports of soaring HMO profits (sometimes exaggerated) and multimillion-dollar executive compensation schemes (usually not exaggerated) compounded the concerns. In fact, those profits were at times pretty skimpy. By one estimate, 40 percent of HMOs lost money in 1995 and only 35 percent were profitable in 1996 (Center for Studying Health System Change, 1997). Indeed, in the last quarter of 1996, HMO profits, on average, were in the red (Hilzenrath, July 1997).

But pleas of poverty from the managed care industry have fallen on deaf consumer ears. What the consumer is likely to hear and remember is that Foundation Health Plan executive Dan Crowley made $19 million in one year or that HealthSource Corporation's Richard Scrushy received $11.4 million in 1996.

Percent of Managed Care Enrollees in For-profit Plans

1983	20% of HMO members
1997	62% of HMO members
1997	90% of PPO members

Source: AAHP, Interstudy.

They may have read that leaders of the nation's largest health care companies received pay boosts averaging over 25 percent in 1996 ("Healthcare CEO Compensation Jumped 25%," 1997). One has to almost pity the managed care public relations employee required to explain that his CEO deserved a multimillion-dollar compensation package because he had discovered how to raise corporate profits by delivering fewer services to consumers.

It is hard to guess where this concern will lead. Many Americans generally support markets as the best way to improve goods and services. They might also recognize that multimillion-dollar incomes for corporate executives are not unique to the health care industry. Making money in America is no crime. Issues of monopoly notwithstanding, profitmaking is presumed to result from providing more value—producing a better product or service at the same or lower price. That should be no different in health care than in other economic sectors.

But beyond the theory, the managed care organization has trouble here. CEOs of Disney, McDonalds, or Microsoft are perceived to be generating profit by giving consumers more—not less. So it is not hard to see why many consumers view their needs for choice, access, and quality as being squeezed between the desire of employers to pay less and the desire of increasingly distant and profit-driven managed care organizations to do less and make more. Greater state scrutiny of plan and hospital conversions and forced disclosure of "medical loss ratios"—the percentage of plan funds expended on medical care, as opposed to administration or profit—are two alternative approaches aimed at this set of issues.

THE PHYSICIAN BACKLASH

The effect of managed care on the health care consumer is the main focus of this chapter, and indeed of this book. But it would be a mistake to forget just how profoundly managed care has affected doctors and the work they do. It is hard enough for most nonphysicians to imagine what it means to devote seven or more prime years of life to the grueling self-sacrifice it takes to become a practicing doctor. Then, consider what it would feel like if the professional world you discovered upon arrival was radically different from what you had been promised. Your income is not what you had projected when you got your student loans, and your hours are longer than you had promised your family.

Perhaps most disheartening of all, while most people get graduate degrees in order to achieve positions that offer some autonomy and even authority, as a managed care physician you may subject yourself to the decisions of a nondoctor on the other end of a phone line and be immersed in red tape more oppressive than your worst nightmare. You may not be able to prescribe the drug you think best for treatment because it is not on the formulary of the health plan of the patient in need. You may be reluctant to refer a patient to a specialist you trust because that doctor is not on the HMO's panel. In one case, author Berenson had to justify a continued stay in the hospital for a critically ill patient with cirrhosis of the liver to seven different HMO nurses and physicians over a two-week period. (That the patient died in the hospital suggests that the need for the continued stay was, indeed, justified).

As we saw in Chapter 3, physicians have been resisting managed care since the beginning. But where once they fought from a position of power, many now feel as if their camp has been overrun. More than a few have quit the profession out of frustration. Others have become politically active to a degree they never imagined, lobbying for legislative restrictions on managed care's power to "practice medicine" or talking about forming unions. And most important, doctors frequently let their frustrations show to patients, no doubt fomenting much of the consumer discontent explored in this chapter.

As a result, managed care has forged a new kind of bond between practitioner and patient—one that has made some strange political bedfellows. Their fears and needs can bring them together. The fight for physician autonomy and patient concerns about the loss of a patient-first ethic go hand in hand. The result can be a lobbying alliance of traditionally conservative physician organizations and traditionally liberal consumer groups—opposing gag clauses and asserting the values of patient choice, even the rights of physicians to participate in managed care networks.

That said, there is a lot to be skeptical about in the physicians' critique. We would like to think of doctors as a source of authoritative commentary about managed care's effect on quality. After all, who is in a better position to assess the impact of managed care policies and operations than those clinicians whose behavior managed care directly affects? Who better to expose the difference between slick advertising about a plan's commitment to improving quality and the reality as seen in specific policies that directly affect the quality of care patients are receiving? And yet the purchasers of health care have virtually ignored the opinions of medical associations that are critical of managed care. Indeed, some purchasers conclude that a managed care plan cannot be doing a good job if physicians in its network are not complaining. Managed care organizations known among physicians as "doctor-friendly" can actually lose business because employers are concerned that if physicians consider the program to be friendly to them, the physicians must have too much influence on it. The result, purchasers fear, will be an inability of the plan to hold down costs.

Unfortunately, purchasers' instincts in this regard may not be too far off the mark. Physicians often have a difficult time separating their self-interest from the best interests of their patients. They of course insist that, above all, the new environment is a threat to patients and that patients are their first consideration. But, their substantial incomes notwithstanding, many physician attacks on the very logic of managed care are often far off target and far too one-sided.

Let us consider the autonomy issue. Without question, many preauthorization programs are demeaning and poorly conceived. But utilization management, as we have tried to show, can also be effective both in controlling costs and improving quality. Patients can receive more evidence-based, coordinated care, and physicians can learn new ways to improve their ability to care for patients. As a result, physician attacks on utilization management can often appear more like efforts to reassert the old blank-check system than legitimate and measured critiques. Physician attacks on gag clauses have also been misleading, suggesting that the problem is much larger than it is. And physician support of "any willing provider" rules that would give them rights to participate in networks, while also expressed in terms of public needs, clearly have physician benefit written all over them.

Today, physicians find themselves with much less influence over managed care than they would like and much less than they should have. But the situation is, at least in part, their own doing. In the worst case, their situation is akin to the boy who cried wolf once too often and was then swallowed up because others stopped listening.

Fortunately, increasing numbers of physicians and physician groups are now focused more on improving managed care than undermining it. At minimum, they have accepted the need to add factors of cost into the medical equation and have recognized the values of improved communication and coordination among physicians and between physicians and other health professionals; at maximum, they are seeking to lead managed care organizations in the search for improved quality.

CONCLUSION: CONSUMERS AT RISK

Managed care companies may well decry today's media critique of their industry as based too heavily on anecdote. But to deny the legitimacy of consumer concerns about managed care would be absurd. Managed care strategies, when wisely implemented, may hold great potential for improving the quality of American health care. But, as we have argued earlier, those same strategies implemented less conscientiously can pose real threats to that quality. Good organization is almost certainly better than no organization. But bad organization may be worst of all.

This is not to suggest that the wave of proconsumer or anti-managed care legislation is all justified. We will argue that much of it is not. Indeed, we will argue that much of that legislative response, as well as certain marketplace demands being made by consumers today, misses the consumer protection mark. Some elements of that agenda may actually undermine the drive for higher quality health care.

7

The Managed Care Record: Better Than You Think

Sympathy for the Devil

On June 30, 1997, the *Washington Post* ran a front-page story entitled "Backlash Builds over Managed Care. Frustrated Consumers Push for Tougher Laws." The article detailed deep anxiety over managed care and how most state legislatures and state government officials felt the need to respond. On the very same day, the *Wall Street Journal* ran a front-page story, "Health-Cost Trims Hold Inflation Down." This piece attributed the broad move to managed care as a primary reason for the current economic expansion and low rate of inflation in the country and wondered whether managed care's success can be sustained.

Together, these stories suggest some causes of the current skepticism about managed care. It has been relatively easy to arouse public concern with stories of individual people misused by the new system. It has been much more difficult for Americans to recognize the benefits managed care has produced.

This contrast should help us better understand the other side of the consumer backlash against managed care, which can reflect misunderstanding, exaggeration, and distortion of both the past and the present. Moreover, focusing as it has on regulatory approaches to preventing managed care organizations from doing harm to individuals, our dominant social and political discussion about managed care may be ignoring opportunities to push plans to improve care for all. As a result, our failure to rationally assess the strengths and weaknesses of managed care could easily undermine the overall pursuit of high-quality care at an affordable price.

In this chapter, we will look at the potential flaws in the anti-managed care case outlined in Chapter 6. Many of these we have already discussed and only require mention here. Once having reviewed this side of the argument, we will look at the best evidence available on quality in managed care. Our assessment will lead us to the questions of what should and should not be done, and who might or might not do it.

IT COSTS LESS, AND THAT COUNTS

It is impossible to project exactly what health care costs would be today if the old system of fee-for-service had stayed intact. But it is safe to say that employers and employees today would be paying at least 10 percent and perhaps as much as 50 percent more for the same benefits packages. In fact, two California analysts projected that if 1988–1992 trends continued through 1997, health insurance premiums for California state employees would be twice what they are today, at a cost to taxpayers and employees of $1.5 billion per year (Enthovan, Singer, 1997).

Consumers acknowledge that managed care saves money. But they tend to think the savings have gone to employers and insurers, not to them—and to some extent they are right. While premiums paid by employers have risen little over the last five years, employers have been shifting more of those premium costs to employees. This has been especially true for premiums paid for individuals as opposed to those for families, with many employees paying as much as twice as much in 1996 as they did in 1988 (Gabel, Ginsburg, and Hunt, 1997). In any case, without seeing themselves as the beneficiaries of managed care, consumers are less likely to see its value and less likely to accept its restrictions as acceptable trade-offs.

The same reluctance to accept the cost trade-off may be at work in today's managed care regulation debate. Many of the consumer-protection proposals now before state and federal legislatures would certainly increase costs. Laws guaranteeing rights to longer hospital stays increase costs. So too would laws requiring all plans to offer a POS option or guaranteed access to certain specialists. So too would laws restricting the means by which plans pay providers, or laws that guaranteed physicians more rights to participation in networks. The perceived benefits of such laws may or may not be worth the costs. But the trade-off needs to be acknowledged and the costs counted.

Critics of managed care might be wise to ask: if health care costs had to come down (and they did), what would cost control have been like under the fee-for-service system? That system, it should be remembered, had no means of improving efficiency or reducing unnecessary or inappropriate care. Its only means of lowering costs and premiums were to deny payment for services or to reduce payments to physicians and hospitals, who would then collect the difference from patients. If these approaches did not work, employers could reduce the benefits they offered or stop buying insurance altogether.

Consumers would be the losers in each of these scenarios. Viewed from this perspective, trade-offs imposed by managed care may not look so bad. Employers, government, and even society at large were demanding that health care costs come down. Someone, somehow, had to do the dirty work.

BLAME THE SYSTEM

Concerns about managed care sometimes result from a tendency to blame the system precisely because there is a system, whether or not it is to blame. Consider, for example, the following case.

In treating Ms. Simpson, who has a conventional fee-for-service insurance plan, Dr. Jones makes a mistake. She fails to recognize the symptoms of angina pectoris, and thus fails to recognize that Ms. Simpson needs to see a cardiologist. Three weeks later, Ms. Simpson suffers a heart attack and dies. If the mistake is recognized, the family may blame Dr. Jones. They may even sue her. But the finger-pointing probably stops there. There is no "system" to blame for this error.

Contrast that scenario with one in which Dr. Jones is a member of group practice and Ms. Simpson an enrollee in an HMO that pays Dr. Jones's medical group a fixed amount per month for treating Ms. Simpson and other HMO members. Dr. Jones makes the same mistake with the same unfortunate outcome. But now the outcome may be viewed differently. Dr.

Jones's failure to refer Ms. Simpson could be portrayed as stemming from financial incentives applied by the group or HMO. Ms. Simpson's lawyers would argue that she did not get referred because it would cost Dr. Jones and her colleagues money. Thus, the medical group and the HMO, not simply Dr. Jones, come to be blamed. From there, it is a short step to blaming managed care in general. In a worst-case scenario, the story will appear on page one of the local paper as another HMO horror story (see figure below).

Critics of managed care are right, of course, to be wary of potential systemic failures. But they should also consider how the absence of systems can lead to mistakes and failure and how good systems might prevent them. Many proposals being considered in legislatures today would have the effect of reducing a

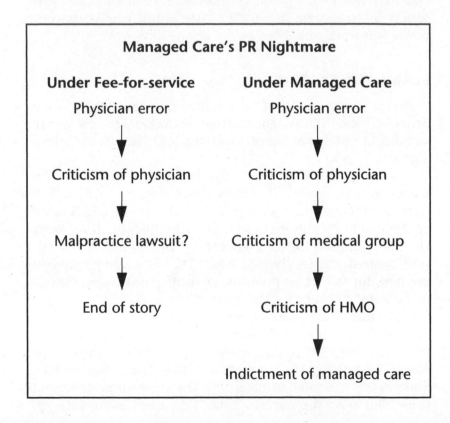

system's control over patient care. All kinds of measures relating to choice and access to out-of-network providers fall into this category. When applied to an irresponsible managed care plan, they offer obvious advantages. But they can also have the effect of undermining the incentives for plans to develop and implement clinical practice guidelines, pursue preventive care approaches, and invest in information systems that improve coordination within the network. It is interesting to note, in this regard, that the managed care plans that tend to receive the highest ratings in reviews by magazines, including *Consumer Reports*, accrediting agencies, and even public opinion polls tend to be those that have achieved the highest levels of integration—often associated with significant restrictions on or penalties for going out of the network (Brink and Shute, 1997; "The State of Quality in Managed Care," 1997).

EXAGGERATED FEARS

The consumer reform or anti-managed care case also suffers from exaggerated fears of how various strategies work and the impacts they may have. For example, on October 7, 1997, the *Washington Post* reported on a poll of physicians. The headline read: "Physicians report inability to make referrals." The headline seemed to reflect a widely expressed concern about managed care—that access to specialists will be inappropriately restricted. The actual poll results, however, reflected a different picture. In fact, 82 percent of responding physicians reported that they could always or almost always obtain the referrals they thought necessary (see figure, page 124). As for patients, 66 percent strongly disagreed with the proposition that their doctor did not refer them to specialists when needed, and another 17 percent disagreed somewhat. In a separate national survey of two thousand physicians, insurance company denial rates for physician recommended services turn out to be much smaller than managed care critics contend. Only 1.0 percent of recommended hospitalizations, 1.2 percent of surgical procedures and 2.6 percent of referrals to specialists of choice were denied (Remler and others, 1997)

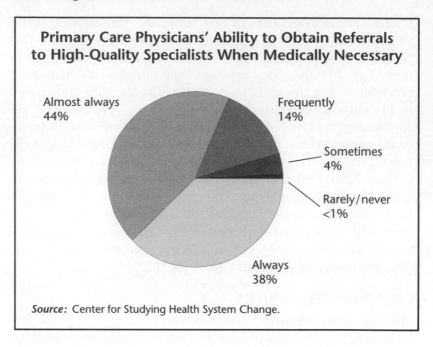

Primary Care Physicians' Ability to Obtain Referrals to High-Quality Specialists When Medically Necessary

Almost always 44%

Frequently 14%

Sometimes 4%

Rarely/never <1%

Always 38%

Source: Center for Studying Health System Change.

The controversy over capitated payments to physicians may offer another example of exaggerated fears. Capitated-payment strategies are certainly on the rise, and the new incentives are gradually changing the way physicians practice medicine. When physicians are "at risk," they become more conservative in their use of resources. They may, for example, be less inclined to order an MRI scan costing hundreds of dollars for a patient with back strain.

But the widespread impression that physicians are at great financial risk for the services they provide is an exaggeration. So, too, are fears that financial pressures are such that physicians are consistently driven to put cost over patient needs. In fact, incomes of physicians do not rise or fall dramatically as the number of referrals they make to specialists or the number of patients they send to the hospital goes up or down. Primary care physicians do not, as some may imagine, take out their personal checkbook every time they refer a patient to a specialist.

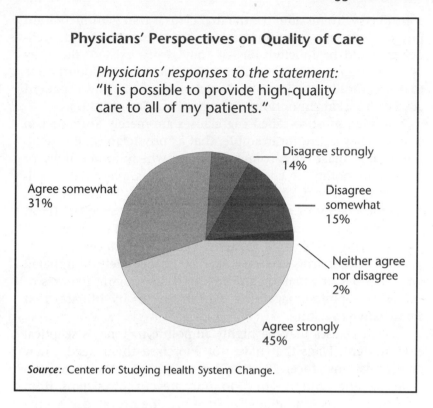

Physicians' Perspectives on Quality of Care

Physicians' responses to the statement:
"It is possible to provide high-quality care to all of my patients."

Disagree strongly
14%

Agree somewhat
31%

Disagree somewhat
15%

Neither agree nor disagree
2%

Agree strongly
45%

Source: Center for Studying Health System Change.

Moreover, capitation payments are much more likely to go to groups than to individuals. In this way, risk is spread over a group of physicians, greatly diffusing whatever pressure an individual doctor might experience. In fact, the individual members of a capitated group may actually receive a salary, with some modest penalties or bonuses attached to encourage prudent use of resources or other values. When we recall that capitation can produce some significant and positive by-products in terms of physician integration and coordination, the strategy looks less alarming and more positive. In the absence of evidence of harm, proposals to place specific limits on the strategy, therefore, seem premature.

Similarly exaggerated are fears that many managed care plans undermine consumer trust by imposing limits on free communication between doctors and patients: the "gag clause" controversy. To be sure, contractual clauses that genuinely limit physician-patient communication about options and well-being would be indefensible—if they really existed. But they don't. Indeed, one analysis of over 700 such clauses found none that specifically restricted a physician from offering a patient advice on treatment options (Etheredge and Jones, 1997).

In fact, most so-called gag clauses are merely anticriticism clauses. They assert, for example, that a "physician shall take no action nor make any communication which undermines or could undermine the confidence of enrollees, potential enrollees, their employers, plan sponsors or the public in Choice Care, or in the quality of care Choice Care enrollees receive" (Pear, 1996). Similar clauses note that "the [HMO] and provider shall portray each other in a positive light to enrollees and the public" or that "this contract may be immediately terminated for . . . provider's making any repeated disparaging remarks or expressing opinions regarding plan or any of its affiliates that are negative in nature."

Such clauses may be highly impolitic in today's skeptical environment. Plans that have not exorcized them need a new public relations officer. But they are not genuine threats to physician-patient candor. They do not prevent physicians from offering patients candid advice. In short, the prevalence of true gag clauses and their significance have frequently been blown out of proportion. The result can be an unjustified level of fear regarding lost candor in managed care relationships.

TOO BROAD A BRUSH

Over time, in a mature, open, and competitive marketplace, those organizations that do not produce value nearly equivalent to that of their competitors will not prosper. Those that cannot produce reasonable blends of price and quality, or that deliver that blend too inconsistently, will be identified. They will have to improve or suffer economic consequences. Purchasers will develop an ability to evaluate the choices available to them and to distinguish between those who produce more value and those who produce less.

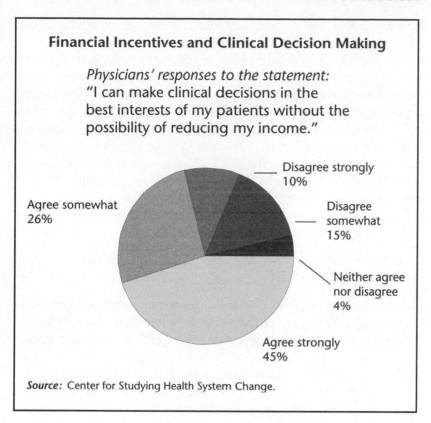

Financial Incentives and Clinical Decision Making

Physicians' responses to the statement:
"I can make clinical decisions in the best interests of my patients without the possibility of reducing my income."

Disagree strongly
10%

Agree somewhat
26%

Disagree somewhat
15%

Neither agree nor disagree
4%

Agree strongly
45%

Source: Center for Studying Health System Change.

But for reasons we will review in greater detail later, the managed care marketplace still lacks these kinds of characteristics. It remains difficult for purchasers to assess the value of the choices available and to distinguish among them. American consumers can distinguish the finest of differences between two cars on the new-car lot. But we have few tools to identify even large differences between managed care plans. As a result, those behaving responsibly can easily get lumped together with those behaving irresponsibly. The anecdote about one HMO denying a patient access to an appropriate but expensive procedure becomes an indictment of managed care in general, not an indictment of *one* managed care plan. This inability to distinguish between the good, the bad, and the ugly is unfortunate not just because it is inaccurate, but because it may reduce both the value of acting responsibly and the danger of acting irresponsibly.

In fact, managed care plans *are* different—not just in how they pay physicians or how much choice they offer. Some are better than others. As the ability to judge and assess their value improves, the differences will become clearer and the bad actors—like bad actors in any marketplace—will find survival more difficult. Until then, however, the temptation to throw the proverbial baby out with the bathwater needs to be resisted. Laws and rules that might seem necessary in restraining a few bad actors, like a law requiring all plans to offer a point-of-service option, may unnecessarily limit the ability of others to improve and innovate.

MISUNDERSTANDING VALUE

Perhaps the most serious weakness in the managed care critique is a failure to see the potential value in some managed care constructs. As a result, some have been too quick to advocate policies that, in the name of consumer protection, might undermine the capacity of some managed care plans to lower costs or raise quality. Here, again, the best example may be the failure to see the potential benefits of capitation and physician risk sharing. In addition to encouraging coordination among physicians, the acceptance of risk is likely to make physicians more committed to improving the physician enterprise and its services. And while there may be concerns about physician-patient trust when cost control becomes the physician's responsibility, capitation does deliver control over the patient's health care back to physicians, removing it from insurers and the intrusive cost-control mechanisms they would otherwise have to impose. One wonders, in this regard, how most consumers would answer the following question: Assuming that the effort to control costs means that someone has to make some rules regarding the use of medical services, should it be your insurer or your physician? We suspect most would choose their physician.

When imposed responsibly, in other words, capitation provides the mechanism for physicians to take back some of their lost control over medical decision making—not under the outmoded professional model, but under a market model that requires accountability for both cost and quality. Those who contemplate reducing the "threats" posed by capitation, then, should be careful not to eliminate the opportunities as well.

Many of the same kinds of risks to innovation and improvement are involved in other anti-managed care legislation. Limiting how plans structure choices, trade-offs, network arrangements, and so on can all sound proconsumer. But they may come with expensive price tags.

QUALITY IN MANAGED CARE: WHAT WE KNOW AND DON'T KNOW

Harold Luft is a health policy researcher at the University of California, San Francisco Medical Center, who has been assessing managed care for nearly two decades. Over that time, he and his colleagues have published three articles summarizing the findings of studies comparing managed care and conventional insurance. Among other things, they review data on the use of services, spending, quality of care, and patient satisfaction. They use the strictest of criteria in deciding what studies to include in their reviews.

In a 1994 review, Luft and his colleague Robert Miller concluded that HMO plan enrollees consistently received more preventive tests, procedures, and examinations, such as cancer and hypertension screening tests, as well as health-promotion activities, such as smoking cessation counseling, than did fee-for-service enrollees (Miller and Luft, 1994). In all but two of sixteen quality-related studies they reviewed, quality of care in HMOs was as good or better than in conventional insurance plans. These included a number of studies focused specifically on individuals in Medicare. Significantly, the two studies that indicated better quality under conventional insurance were both related to care of patients with mental health problems.

In their 1997 update covering studies conducted subsequent to their 1994 review, Miller and Luft appeared to reach a somewhat more cautious conclusion regarding quality of care in HMOs. There were, they reported, "equal numbers of statistically significant positive and negative results for HMO performance, compared to non-HMO plans." In other words, the number of cases or measures in which HMOs came out better than non-HMO plans and the number on which they came out worse were the same. The data, then, suggest that HMOs overall may be no worse, but also no better, than other plans. One point of concern, Miller and Luft emphasized, was treatment of chronically ill patients. Several studies and measures on which HMOs faired worse relative to fee-for-service involved these patients[1] (Miller and Luft, 1997).

A similar review of recent studies on quality of care was conducted by Steven Miles and colleagues from the University of Minnesota's Center for Bioethics. Their findings, presented in December 1996, also show little difference between the quality of care in managed care and in fee-for-service. Three studies found virtually no differences in prenatal care, Caesarian section rates, or birth outcomes. A review of five studies focused on hospitals revealed that HMOs may turn to invasive procedures somewhat less frequently for cardiac and other patients in intensive care. But there was no difference in the rates at which patients in the two groups died, suggesting that the less intense use of high-tech procedures did not compromise quality. In

---

1. Luft and Miller are quick to note the many limitations of studies comparing the two systems. They acknowledge, for example, that the continuing evolution in forms of managed care makes comparisons difficult. In the 1970s, virtually all managed care consisted of nonprofit, traditional group practice model HMOs. In the 1980s, the major expansion was in the IPA-model of HMO. By the 1990s, most of the expansion was in for-profit IPA-HMOs and PPOs and the newer point-of-service products. Studies drawing conclusions about one form of managed care may not be relevant to other forms. Data collection in such studies can go on for years, even as plans change in form and operation. Not all plans are open to such studies, and there is a possibility that those that are may feel they have less to hide. Luft and Miller also recognize that even the most recent studies are based on data that is a few years old and may not reflect some of the most recent and aggressive cost-cutting efforts in managed care.

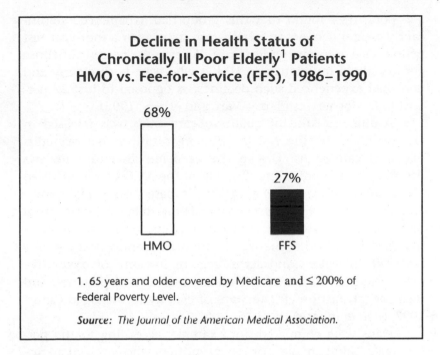

**Decline in Health Status of
Chronically Ill Poor Elderly[1] Patients
HMO vs. Fee-for-Service (FFS), 1986–1990**

68%

27%

HMO   FFS

1. 65 years and older covered by Medicare and ≤ 200% of
Federal Poverty Level.

Source: The Journal of the American Medical Association.

seven studies examining care for elderly patients, Medicare beneficiaries in HMOs did about as well as those in traditional
Medicare on most quality-related criteria. HMOs tended to
emphasize regular examination and preventive services more
than fee-for-service plans. Medicare fee-for-service patients were
more likely to see specialists than were HMO enrollees, although
it was not established that such increased access resulted in
improved quality.

Certainly, as noted in each of these reviews, there is some
reason to be concerned about how managed care may be faring
with certain vulnerable populations. In one study of chronically
ill patients published in 1996, for example, researchers at the
Health Institute of the New England Medical Center found that
physical and mental health outcomes for chronically ill patients
were, as a whole, similar in HMO and fee-for-service settings
(Ware, 1996). But when researchers looked specifically at the
subgroup of chronically ill individuals who were both elderly

and poor, they found that this group had experienced significantly greater declines in health care status over a four-year test period. (See accompanying figure.) Sixty-eight percent of those chronically ill individuals in HMOs who were both elderly and poor had experienced such declines, as opposed to just 27 percent in fee-for-service plans (Ware and others, 1996).

A different kind of quality-of-care study was released in October 1997 by the NCQA, the organization that accredits managed care plans. Unlike the academic literature reviews described in the preceding discussion, the NCQA's report titled *The State of Managed Care Quality* is based on performance, accreditation, and consumer-satisfaction data collected from 329 HMOs and other managed care plans. Its main theme is that HMOs and other managed care organizations *"vary greatly both within regions and across regions in terms of preventive care, treatment of acutely ill and chronically ill patients, and member satisfaction"* ("The State of Quality in Managed Care," 1997, their emphasis).

Plans were compared, for example, according to the percentage of adult smokers or recent quitters who received advice from their plans about how to stop. The average plan score was 61 percent, but scores ranged from a low of 30 percent to a high of 85 percent. Differences between plans on the use of beta-blocker treatment after a heart attack were just as large. Commented NCQA president Margaret O'Kane: "Study after study has shown that treating heart attack patients with beta blockers saves lives, but in some plans, fewer than 30 percent of such patients receive them while in others more than 90 percent do; the patients lost in the gap between what is achievable and what we actually achieve are at greatly increased risk for another heart attack and even death" (NCQA press release, 1997). Similar differences were found in other measures, including breast cancer screening, childhood immunizations, and eye examinations for patients with diabetes.

The NCQA study also concluded that on all the performance measures it reviewed, "the performance of managed care plans is as good or better than that of fee-for-service insurers." They were quick to note, however, that such comparisons are

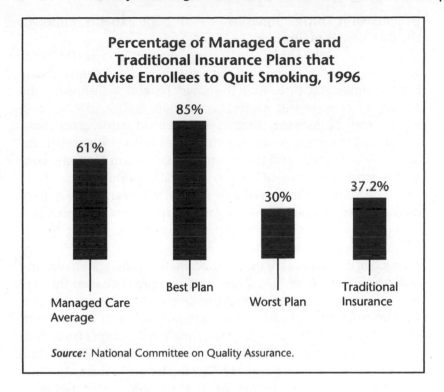

**Percentage of Managed Care and
Traditional Insurance Plans that
Advise Enrollees to Quit Smoking, 1996**

85%

61%

37.2%

30%

Best Plan

Managed Care
Average

Worst Plan

Traditional
Insurance

Source: National Committee on Quality Assurance.

difficult to make and that "conclusions about the overall quality
of managed care vs. fee-for-service cannot be drawn yet" ("The
State of Quality in Managed Care," 1997).

We outline these findings in some detail because they offer
the best information available on the quality of care being delivered in managed care today. For our purposes here, several conclusions stand out.

First, the studies do not support the fears of many managed care critics. There is no evidence of an epidemic of shoddy
care compromising the health and well-being of patients in
HMOs, the form of managed care about which most concern is
expressed. Overall, HMOs appear to deliver about the same quality of care as conventional plans. They may provide higher quality to generally healthy populations, largely because of their
emphasis on prevention. But they may not do quite as well with

patients with chronic illnesses or with poor patients, although the data here is preliminary.

Second, if the studies do not support the fears of HMO critics, neither do they support the case of HMO defenders. The logic of managed care, that it should be able to improve the quality of care, is still more theory than reality. HMOs, as a whole, may be proving themselves to be no worse than traditional fee-for-service plans. But they have not yet demonstrated that they are better, and there is particular reason for some concern regarding the care offered to vulnerable populations.

The failure of managed care to improve health care quality might not be troublesome if, in fact the quality of care provided Americans was consistently high. But it is not. Robert Brook, M.D., Professor of Medicine at UCLA and a prominent researcher in health care quality succinctly sums up what many now know to be true: ". . . There are large gaps between the care that people should receive and the care they do receive. . . It is true in different types of health care facilities and for different types of health insurance. It's true for all age groups, from children to the elderly. And it is true whether one is looking at the whole country or at any one city" (Schuster and others, 1997).

Third, although quality of care probably does not vary much between different conventional insurance plans—all they really do is pay the bills, after all—the same is not true of managed care plans, especially HMOs. The organization that managed care brings to health care delivery has the potential to improve quality, but the potential is not always achieved. As a result, some plans are much better than others. As Miller and Luft conclude, "The results show something that is simple, obvious, and yet sometimes underemphasized: HMOs produce better, the same, and worse quality of care, depending on the particular organization and particular disease" (Miller and Luft, 1997).

CONSUMER SATISFACTION

A considerable amount of research has been done on consumer satisfaction in managed care versus non-managed care plans. It tends to show that satisfaction levels in traditional plans is sometimes higher, but also that it is reasonably high in both types of insurance. We find both conclusions to be of only modest significance.

It might be expected that consumers in conventional plans would be more satisfied. They have full choice of physician and face fewer restrictions on access. The finding of high levels of satisfaction in both types of plans should also be expected. The great majority of enrollees in all plans are healthy and have little occasion to contact their plan. They should have little reason to be "dissatisfied." Indeed, at least one survey has documented that those with better health status tend to be more satisfied with their health plans (Ullman, 1997).

This is not to suggest that comparisons of satisfaction levels in different managed care plans might not be of value and significance to consumers. Especially as these surveys become more sophisticated and begin to focus more—as they should—on those who have had more medical problems and thus more contact with their health plan, their value should increase. Our only point here is that comparisons between satisfaction levels in managed care and non-managed care plans probably do not yet tell us a great deal.

QUALITY IN MANAGED CARE: THEY'RE BOTH WRONG

In summary, when it comes to evaluating managed care today, both the critics and the defenders are wrong. Critics raise legitimate concerns, some of which may need to be addressed by government. But their analysis is often flawed by exaggerated fears of poor quality, reluctance to acknowledge managed care's accomplishments in lowering costs, and a failure to recognize the potential of managed care to improve quality. Moreover, the hard evidence that does exist does not support their worst fears.

However, managed care's defenders often fail to acknowledge that the strength of managed care still lies more in its logic than its practice. Some plans probably do offer very high-quality care; some offer much less than that; and there may be some serious weak links, specifically the quality of care offered to those who are most vulnerable. Overall, HMOs and other managed care organizations have not clearly demonstrated that they can provide better quality care than that provided under the old fee-for-service system. And that is not saying much. Moreover, as we have suggested earlier, there are some trends afoot that can threaten the overall level of quality now provided in managed care.

The central questions, then, are: Why isn't managed care achieving its potential to improve quality and what can be done about it? In Chapter 8 we will look at the first question, and in Chapters 9 and 10 we will address the second.

8

Rule of Price; Cult of Choice; Cost of Quality

You Better Shop Around

As outlined in the preceding chapters, the old system of fee-for-service medicine was not nearly as good as many think. It failed both to control costs and to promote higher quality. When compared to the old system, the logic of managed care is compelling, in terms of potential for lowering cost and for raising quality. Public concern over managed care arrangements is understandable, but the current critique of managed care is also seriously flawed. Overall, managed care has led to lower health care costs and has produced a quality of care that is at least equal to that produced in the old fee-for-service system. But there is little evidence that managed care is improving the quality of care delivered or the health status of Americans. In short, it is not living up to its logic or potential.

The biggest disappointment in managed care, then, may not be what it is, but what it isn't. Moreover, there is reason to be concerned that, if certain marketplace trends continue, quality of care in many managed care arrangements could be threatened. Why is managed care failing to achieve its potential to raise quality, and what can be done about it?

THE COMPONENTS OF VALUE

It is common these days to hear about efforts to cultivate "value-based purchasing" in health care. Purchasers proudly proclaim that they are evaluating health plans based on both the quality they offer and the price they charge. That, in itself, is a startling admission. In purchasing just about anything, don't we always look at price, quality, and the relationship between the two, that is, at value?

The answer, of course, is yes for almost all things, but not always for health care. In the fee-for-service world, the two core attributes of value—price and quality—were treated uniquely. Price was not as important as it was with other products, because it was often hidden and passed through. Even if purchasers did want to choose a plan based on price, there was not much to choose from or compare: virtually all insurance plans paid all providers, and most agreed to pay 80 percent of what providers charged, so they could not do much to control their price.[1] Quality, meanwhile, was assumed to reside in the individual providers chosen, not in the insurance plan. For health plans, then, quality was not an issue.

But in the new managed care marketplace all that has changed. The strategies and tools of managed care are capable of affecting both price and quality. Competition can now exist, theoretically at least, on both. Value-based purchasing has become possible.

But today's value-based purchasing seems out of balance and far from ideal. Three realities stand out. First, price and quality have nowhere near equal weight. Price is of utmost concern to employer/purchasers, who feel they have been paying too much for too long. Second, quality is hard to define, demonstrate, and market. Third, in the absence of proven quality and given public concerns over restrictions in managed care, choice of physician has become the public's safety net and a proxy for quality. The result has been a marketplace dynamic featuring aggressive competition on price and expanding net-

---

1. In fact, especially as traditional insurers began to experience competition from managed care organizations, traditional insurers began employing utilization management to control costs. Many plans would pay providers less than 80 percent of their charges, claiming that the provider charged more than the "usual and customary" amount. The physician would then have to seek any additional payment from the consumer. But, overall, providers set their prices, insurers paid 80 percent, and there was not too much insurers did or could do to control the price.

works that accommodate the demand for greater choice. Quality is more often the subject of lip service than serious attention.

PRICE: THE BOTTOM LINE RULES

Tongue-in-cheek, Princeton University economist Uwe Reinhardt describes the uniqueness of the old health marketplace rules. Each year, he explains, he would ask his freshman economics students what happens to price when there is an excess of supply. Surprisingly, he found, there were always a few students who got it wrong, thinking that an excess supply would actually push prices up. Perplexed by this inability of Princeton freshmen to understand the simplest of economic realities, Reinhardt probed deeper. Finally the explanation emerged: the students who thought greater supply led to higher prices were all children of doctors (Reinhardt, 1997).

The Quickest Route to Higher Value

Managed care changed the old rules. Suppliers of services were no longer in control. Managed care plans began to compete for employer business. That meant getting cost and price down, and given the bloated nature of the old system, it was not difficult. Patients went to hospitals less frequently and had shorter stays there. Procedures were shifted from expensive hospitals to less expensive out-patient settings. Referrals to specialists declined. And most important, the oversupply of doctors (especially specialists) and hospitals began to produce what oversupply means in most industries: a price-cutting opportunity. Plans began to demand big discounts, and providers had to go along or lose the business.

As they watched and encouraged new levels of competition, employers grew more aware that competition among managed care plans was finally putting them in the driver's seat. They grew more insistent in their demands, and price competition flourished. Competition on quality, by contrast, was a different story. Quality improvement can be harder to achieve and less tangible if achieved. As a result, in spite of all the increased talk about value-based purchasing, virtually everyone who has studied changing health care markets today reports that most employers are focused mostly on price. Employers, they say repeatedly, are extremely "price sensitive."

Surveys confirm this perception. A survey of 1,100 benefits managers, for example, found that cost to the company was the most important factor in choosing health plans. A 1997 survey of employers of over 3,000 individuals found that 86 percent believed cost to be extremely important or very important in their decision to offer HMOs; the second ranking factor, member satisfaction, scored just 69 percent. And on a survey of health plans on factors considered to be important in the marketplace, price was again the clear winner, with 69 percent of plans ranking it first or second. Fifty percent of plans ranked patient satisfaction first or second; just 20 percent ranked quality improvement first or second (McLaughlin, 1997).

Employees, interestingly, view things differently. They tend to rank quality, choice, and benefits over cost—in part, we presume, because they are not paying most of the bill. In a 1996 poll, for example, 42 percent of employees ranked high quality as their most important concern, with "keeps cost low" at just 18 percent (McLaughlin, 1997). Such findings suggest that plans might have more incentive to improve and compete on quality if employees rather than employers were making health plan choices. But, that is not the case today.

Mergers and Marketplace Change

The dominance of price can also be seen in the furious pace of merger and acquisition activity that has distinguished the health care marketplace in recent years. Theoretically, at least, marketplace reorganization and higher quality could go hand in hand. Mergers could create economies of scale that would, for example, enable plans and hospitals to install improved information systems, to move patient information around the country via computer modems, and to smooth the introduction of practice guidelines, as well as enable plans to better track outcomes of various medical interventions.

Thus far, however, the potential of merged organizations to achieve higher quality remains largely untapped. While quality improvement is always accorded much lip service, the focus of most mergers or acquisitions is on securing control over managed care revenue flows and market power, defined as increasing leverage over those from whom one purchases and over those to whom one sells. To Wall Street financiers, this may be about raising revenues and profits by raising market share. In terms of increasing value by raising quality or lowering price, it is mostly about lowering price.

All of this could change, of course. The capacity to collect and compare plans on quality is improving, and those efforts are becoming more public. But the combination of a capacity to lower price, the employer choice, and employer sensitivity to price and intangible nature of improved quality, makes the drive to compete primarily on price almost irresistible. Moreover, if plans feel squeezed by employers resisting higher premiums, some may respond in ways that threaten quality. At some point, exploitation of excess capacity and extensions of market power will not be enough. The only way to hold down price may be to cut quality, deny access, or reduce benefits.

CHOICE: OF PHYSICIAN, PLAN, AND OTHER THINGS

As employers have seized upon managed care to lower price, employees have fretted over the loss of choice—specifically over the loss of choice of physician. If any one issue leaps out from the mass of consumer backlash demands, it is the fear that we may not be able to see our physician of choice. This should not surprise us. In the absence of clear evidence that the new system, including limited physician networks, offers high quality, it is only natural that consumers would fall back on this hallmark of the old system.

Choice of Physician: The New Safety Net

As a result of these demands, the new managed care market-place is exhibiting a dramatic trend toward increasing choice of provider. The trend has come in two broad forms. First, there is the rise (and survival) of managed care forms that offer consumers more out-of-network options, especially point-of-service (POS) plans and PPOs. Just a few years ago, most analysts envisioned the growth of highly integrated systems, with looser arrangements like PPOs proving to be little more than a transition stage from the old system to the new. But those expectations turned out to be far off the mark. PPO and POS plans are here to stay.

> ## The Cult of Choice:
> ## Average Number of Doctors in HMO Networks
>
> 1994   2,124 MDs
>
> 1995   2,660 MDs
>
> % Increase: 24
>
> *Source:* Advisory Board Company.

The second trend has been toward ever broader networks of physicians and hospitals, with most providers in many, if not all, networks. Insurer brochures trumpet that they have over 75 percent of local physicians and hospitals in their networks. "Welcome to the PPO network," wrote one plan to its physicians. "You are now part of a carefully selected panel of more than 300 hospitals and 21,000 physicians" (Berenson, 1997).

Today the biggest and broadest networks may offer the most appeal and, significantly, the quickest means to increasing numbers of enrollees, revenues, and profits. In the view of the Washington-based Advisory Board, a prominent consulting group, "Emerging competition among HMOs [is] centered on breadth of physician and hospital choice; plans in some markets

[are] racing to add providers faster than their competitors to gain an advantage in attracting enrollment" (Health Care Advisory Board, 1995). In what they call the "Battle for New York City," the Advisory Board reports that between 1992 and 1994 Oxford Health Plan expanded the number of physicians in its network from 5,400 to 11,120. During the same period, new enrollments increased from 9,000 in 1992 to 288,584 in 1994. By contrast, competitor U.S. Healthcare expanded its network by just 2,000 physicians in the same period, from 4,282 to 6,194. New annual enrollment grew by less than 10,000 enrollees, from 75,266 to 84,269 (Health Care Advisory Board, 1995).

In the wake of these trends, even the traditional group practice HMOs are changing their ways. The Kaiser system, for example, long an exemplar of the highly integrated system, is introducing PPO and POS plans and contracting with increasing numbers of independent physicians. Kaiser's Northern California plan introduced a PPO in 1994 and a POS plan in 1995, and now contracts with thousands of non-Kaiser physicians and 110 non-Kaiser hospitals. In Southern California, Kaiser members can now visit any physician in that part of the state (Health Care Advisory Board, 1995). Kaiser CEO David Lawrence summed up the current reality: "In recent years there has been a steady drumbeat of companies telling us that they won't offer Kaiser to their employees or that they are dropping us because Kaiser restricts employees to Kaiser doctors and facilities" (Health Care Advisory Board, 1995, as quoted in Integrated Healthcare Report).

Indeed, these developments tempt one to suggest that the most striking trend in managed care today is back to the old system of every doctor in, or at least available in, every plan. This, of course, prompts a question: Will this drive to produce huge networks reduce the ability of plans to hold down costs? The answer is unclear, almost certainly.

On the one hand, some managed care plans have deployed the various tools of managed care to hold down costs even as they expand networks. Many physicians and hospitals remain insecure about being cut out of networks and thus are still prepared to offer deep discounts as a price of inclusion. And

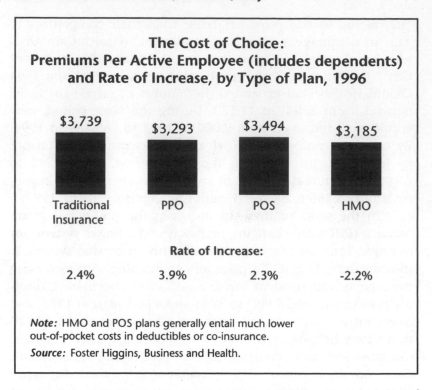

The Cost of Choice:
Premiums Per Active Employee (includes dependents)
and Rate of Increase, by Type of Plan, 1996

$3,739	$3,293	$3,494	$3,185
Traditional Insurance	PPO	POS	HMO

Rate of Increase:

2.4%	3.9%	2.3%	-2.2%

Note: HMO and POS plans generally entail much lower out-of-pocket costs in deductibles or co-insurance.

Source: Foster Higgins, Business and Health.

because they pass some of their higher costs on to employees in the form of more out-of-pocket costs, POS plans and PPOs have been able to hold down their premiums. In these ways, the new managed care marketplace has been able to accommodate both demands of employers for lower price and of consumers for more choice.

On the other hand, there is the example of Oxford Health Plan. Oxford's growth has been explosive, reaching 2 million enrollees by late 1997, with half of them joining since early 1996. Its strategy has been to give consumers what they want—a huge network and easier access to specialists and providers, from New York's prestigious academic medical centers to chiropractors—and all at an HMO price. But by December 1997, Oxford was on the economic ropes. Physicians were complaining of late payment; debts were mounting; and sizable premium increases were anticipated (Abelson, 1997). Where such troubles exist, of course, Wall Street cannot be far behind. Between July 18 and

December 12, 1997, Oxford stock plummeted from almost $86 to $16 a share. Oxford's predicament may have had several causes. But certainly, giving consumers all they wanted at a competitive HMO price was proving difficult, if not impossible. In other words, choice and low price could be on a collision course.

The demand for choice may produce other problems, beyond its potential clash with lower price. Choice of physician and quality are likely to conflict as well. For one thing, expansion of provider choice may undermine the budding drive of some employers to seek out quality. Quality would, as in the old system, be dependent on choice of individual physicians, not of systems of care.

Moreover, as PPOs and IPAs expand in size, the concept of a *network* becomes a stretch. When physicians belong to multiple plans, they are committed to few and integrated into none. In the current District of Columbia market, for example, where managed care has a long history, at least ten plans use essentially the same physician networks. Under these circumstances, efforts to truly manage or coordinate care, to enforce guidelines or protocols, to monitor and evaluate physician practice patterns, or to select physicians for their practice of high-quality, cost-effective medicine become almost impossible. The logic and advantages of managed care become elusive or unattainable. The only "tools" available to "manage" care are ratcheting down on prices paid to providers and insurer-driven, aggressive limits on access and service. And once physicians and hospitals recognize that public demand for choice has increased their leverage over plans, a central element of managed care cost control will be undermined. In the worst-case scenario, the new system might not only begin to look like the old one, it might also begin to cost like the old one.

A Different Choice

The rise of broader, looser networks, and the threat to coordinated care that they impose, suggest something critically important: consumers may be focused on the wrong choice. Rather than seeking protection in choice of physician—which may

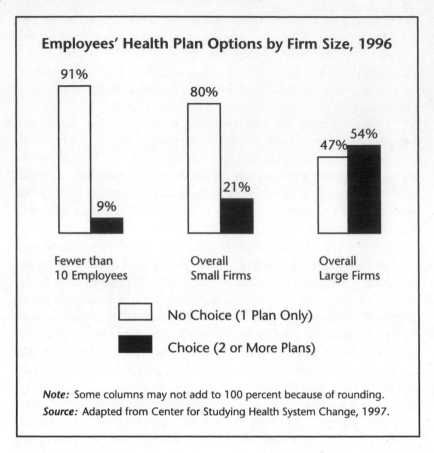

Employees' Health Plan Options by Firm Size, 1996

91%

80%

54%

47%

21%

9%

Fewer than
10 Employees

Overall
Small Firms

Overall
Large Firms

☐ No Choice (1 Plan Only)

■ Choice (2 or More Plans)

Note: Some columns may not add to 100 percent because of rounding.
Source: Adapted from Center for Studying Health System Change, 1997.

move us backwards toward the failures of the old system—consumers might want to think about the values of choice of plan. The latter would offer both protection and a capacity to produce real consumer leverage.

Today, most consumers have little such choice, and trends are toward even less of it. Between 40 and 50 percent of employees have no choice at all. Only 30 percent of employees have a choice of three or more plans, and that number is falling (KPMG employer benefits survey, 1997). Even when the employee does have choice, it is the employer who selects which plans to put on the menu.

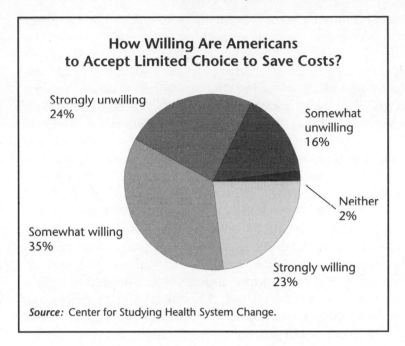

**How Willing Are Americans
to Accept Limited Choice to Save Costs?**

Strongly unwilling
24%

Somewhat
unwilling
16%

Neither
2%

Somewhat willing
35%

Strongly willing
23%

Source: Center for Studying Health System Change.

But plans are different, and choice of plan matters. This is the lesson not just of rigorous academic research and intensive surveys of plans as conducted by organizations like the NCQA, but of such publications as *Consumer Reports*. A *U.S. News and World Report* study published in October 1997 ranked 132 plans in 42 states, comparing them on a host of criteria and then providing an overall evaluation of one to four stars. "The rankings," the report concluded, "have substantial value as a consumer tool. The numbers demonstrate the presence or absence of qualities closely tied to an HMO's quality of care. . . . Given a four-star plan and a three-star plan, it would be hard to argue for the lower-ranked plan unless the scores were close" (*U.S. News and World Report*, October 13, 1997). Hard, indeed, and even harder was the choice between a one-star and a four-star plan.

The value of plan choice can also be seen in the different ways consumers view the trade-off between choice of physician and cost. A 1997 survey conducted for the Center for Studying Health System Change asked consumers how willing they were to accept limited choice of providers in exchange for lower costs. Fifty-eight percent responded that they would be "strongly willing" or "somewhat willing" to accept limited choice to save money. Forty percent said they would be "strongly unwilling" or "somewhat unwilling" to do so. Not surprisingly, those with lower incomes tended to be more willing to accept less choice to get lower price (Center for Studying Health System Change, 1997).

Neither point of view, of course, is right or wrong. We simply want to emphasize that consumers disagree about the trade-off and should have the right to accept the trade-off that best suits their needs. As noted, close to half of Americans in employer-based insurance do not have that option.

As the ability to differentiate between plans—according to style, structure, trade-offs, quality, etc.—grows, the lack of employee choice grows more indefensible. Indeed, employer choice of health plans grew out of historical circumstances, tax policy, and indifference (choice of plan did not matter in the old system), not out of any conscious decision that it was in the best interests of employees. But because their employers are choosing their health plans, Americans may easily find themselves in a plan they do not like or without the option to choose the one they do like. Moreover, leaving a job to start one's own business, losing a job, getting a divorce, or just changing jobs—which the average American does far more often than in the past—can mean having to change plans and maybe doctors as well.

Most important, if individuals had more choice of *plan*, choice of *physician* might seem less critical. If consumers had more choice of plan, they could each decide whether they wanted a plan that allowed them maximum choice of physician; one that was more integrated and structured around a particular medical group, clinic, or hospital system; or something in the middle. They would have much less reason to demand reforms that lock in certain arrangements with regard to physician choice—such as rights to go outside a network or demands that all plans offer some form of point-of-service option. They might even come to view those reforms as restraining rather than increasing their choices and potential trade-offs. Indeed, it may actually be the absence of choice of plan that makes choice of physician seem so critical.

We find it strange, therefore, that American consumers, and even those who try to represent consumers, seem so unconcerned about their lack of choice in plans. Even if they have been somewhat successful in pushing for bigger networks and more choice of physician, American consumers are still allowing their employers to make critical life choices for them.

Choice and the Thing Chosen

The issues of *who* chooses (employer or employee) and *how much* choice there is (of physicians or plans) are compounded by the question of *what* is chosen. Does the purchaser choose an insurer—like United HealthCare, Aetna, or Blue Cross—or a delivery system, medical group, multispecialty clinic, or physician-hospital organization?

In the case of the original group practice HMOs, they were one and the same. Group Health of Puget Sound came with its own exclusive delivery system. But currently, health plans and delivery systems are much more likely to be separate entities, each contracting with many of the other. Thus, today's most common scenario: an employer or employee picks an insurer (e.g., Aetna), who then contracts with individual providers (e.g., Dr. Smith and Dr. Jones), some hospitals, and perhaps one or more delivery systems (e.g., the Mayo Clinic) to deliver care. The insurer may also play a major role in determining how benefits are defined. But increasingly, and especially where capitation is employed, the insurer is less likely to be in control of the actual delivery or quality of care.

But if each plan offers up a loose and diverse network of providers, some of whom overlap with competing plans, how does an employer or employee choose a plan on quality? With difficulty. What the employer or employee may really need to choose, then, is not an insurer, but a specific delivery system.

This could come about in several ways. Delivery systems like the Mayo Clinic, the Henry Ford System in Detroit, or a university health care system could get a license as an insurer and offer themselves directly to employers and individuals. Some have done so. Alternatively, arrangements could be adopted in which employees directly choose not insurers, but delivery systems, which may have ties to insurers, but are not insurers themselves. This is being tried in Minnesota. The Medicare program is also about to experiment with such arrangements.

Another option is the California model. Most providers there have contracts with most of the insurers. Whichever insurer they or their employer chooses, then, the individual consumer is likely to see many if not all of the same providers and provider organizations listed in the network. To this extent, the California market may not be very different from many other markets in which the trend is toward more choice of physician.

But in California, something is different. Increasing numbers of California physicians are connected to large medical groups. These may be structured as traditional group practices or associations of independent practitioners (IPAs) that are likely to be far more integrated than similar associations in other states. Moreover, these medical groups and IPAs, some of which provide only primary care and some of which include specialists, are likely to be capitated by insurers and thus assume full responsibility for the management and delivery of care. So when the consumer chooses a physician, they are really choosing a delivery system that will provide or arrange for all of their health care.

Under this model, the insurer is actually marketing not a loose network of unrelated providers, but a menu of integrated provider systems. In a twist on modern health care terminology, the insurer is acting like a purchasing cooperative, offering individual employees choices of provider-directed delivery systems that have, for most intents and purposes, taken on the functions of an HMO.

In such systems and markets, the focus of competition shifts from insurers, many of which are national in character, to providers and provider systems, almost all of which are locally based. Such competition may be particularly well suited for those interested in seeking higher quality, as it may be easier to assess the quality of a local delivery system than that of a national insurer that contracts with all kinds of provider organizations.

QUALITY: THE STEPCHILD

When price rules, when definitions of choice cut against the grain of quality improvement, and when quality remains hard to define and demonstrate, the search for quality faces an uphill struggle. Getting plans to invest money and energy in quality improvement will be difficult, especially if raising quality means raising price or restricting choice. From a plan or delivery system's point of view, the drive to raise quality may encounter at least four challenges. First, quality must be improved. Second, higher quality must be demonstrable, which means that purchasers must be able to see it and compare it with quality in other systems. Without such a capacity, competition based on quality cannot flourish. Third, once demonstrated, the higher quality must be marketed. Finally, the plan or delivery system may have to live with the reality that better quality can mean higher risk.

Raising Quality

Plan managers or hospital administrators today can look at managed care markets like California, Arizona or Minnesota and see fewer hospital admissions, shorter stays, and the savings that attend them. They can also envision how a new acquisition or merger might provide more market leverage, economies of scale, revenues, and capacity to offer new products. When opportunities like these abound and appear necessary for survival, it can be difficult to get CEOs to focus energy and resources on the less bankable asset of quality improvement.

This is especially true when such improvements are likely to raise costs. Some innovations can indeed raise quality without raising costs; some might even lower costs. A new drug therapy, for example, that reduces the need for a surgical procedure might both raise quality and lower cost. So, too, can a number of prevention strategies. But most plans will adopt such low-cost/ high-quality strategies fairly quickly. Over time, raising and maintaining higher quality than the competition will cost more, just as it does in the case of cars, computers, education, football teams, or just about anything else. For instance, the kinds of computer systems required for maintaining and monitoring patient records, outcomes of care, implementation of sophisti- cated clinical guidelines, and utilization of services by participat- ing providers can cost tens of millions of dollars. To recoup such costs, plans must either increase enrollment or raise prices. If the quality benefits are not compelling and visible, or if price-sensi- tive employers are unwilling to pay a higher price, the case for making the investment sinks.

Efforts to improve quality may also encounter the impera- tive of choice. As we have argued, higher quality is most likely to emerge in more integrated systems. At the HMO level, these systems are likely to be traditional group staff HMO models, many of which routinely achieve the highest scores on perform- ance report cards. At the delivery-system level, the more inte- grated systems tend to be large multispecialty clinics or health systems—like Mayo, Geisinger, Fallon, Scripps, Lovelace, or Intermountain Health Care—or academic medical centers. In other words, quality and integration of services may go together.

But such systems do not offer widespread choice of pro- vider. And they may suffer for it, especially if they are not household names. The benefits of integration may still be largely lost on the general public. Today, at least, the most inte- grated systems are not the clearest of marketplace winners. Thus, again, those interested in doing what seems most likely to maximize quality will need to consider the price they may pay for doing so. If they limit choice and cannot demonstrate and market clearly superior quality—and quickly—they risk market- place losses.

Proving It

Even if an organization can raise its quality, it must demonstrate that improvement and prove its quality superior to others. This has proven exceedingly difficult.

In 1996, General Motors (GM) spent $1,200 per vehicle produced or $4.8 billion on health care coverage for 1.5 million employees and retirees. Each year it engages in a considerable effort to evaluate health plans, to pass the information it gathers on to its employees, and to structure choices for employees that encourage them to pick plans with higher "value." In evaluating plans, GM uses data collected by the NCQA, from other organizations, and from its own surveys. It conducts site visits of plans and consumer-satisfaction surveys to gather feedback from employees. It sets targets and expectations for plans with which it contracts. It then offers its employees a wide choice of plans and scorecard-type information, assigning each choice a "relative plan value." Finally, it makes clear which plans it believes to be the best or "benchmark" plans and tries to encourage enrollment in those plans by paying more of the premium when employees or retirees choose them.

The program produces real results. In 1997, poorly rated plans experienced 50 percent less new enrollment than they had in 1996. The benchmark HMO, by contrast, saw new enrollment grow by over 12 percent (Bradley, 1997).

As the GM experience may indicate, the state of the art in quality assessment is improving. Private employers, employer coalitions, and organizations like the NCQA are developing sophisticated measures of clinical quality and making real progress in forcing insurers to collect and turn over the information necessary to evaluate them. Consumer-satisfaction surveys are also getting more sophisticated. They may not directly reflect medical quality, but as they begin to ask consumers about their health status and how it has changed, rather than about comfort in the waiting room, they will yield more valuable information. Movements are also afoot to standardize them, so that results can be more easily compared.

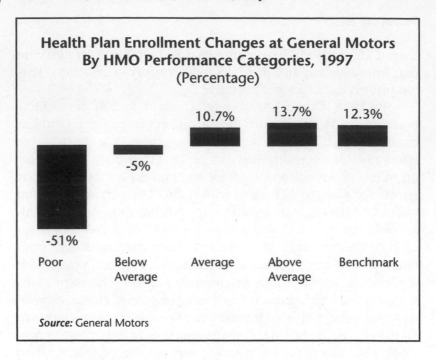

**Health Plan Enrollment Changes at General Motors
By HMO Performance Categories, 1997**
(Percentage)

Source: General Motors

But GM is the exception, not the rule. A review of efforts to evaluate and compare plans on quality leaves one struck more by the complexity and challenge of the task than by successes achieved in it. Frustrations abound. Performance reports such as those developed by the NCQA may not be as revealing as once hoped. Observers note that as soon as a particular performance measure like immunization rates for children under age two is accepted for use, plans begin to focus on that marker like a student studying to pass an exam rather than to get educated. Achieving valid comparisons on actual medical outcomes, such as relief of heart disease, is even more difficult and expensive. Such studies must extend over long periods of time, and researchers must somehow make certain that the outcome achieved was the result of the specific medical intervention undertaken and not of extraneous factors.

Accreditation also has its limitations. Consumers do not know much about what accreditation implies. And Wall Street analysts reportedly give little credit for it (Gabel, 1997). Presumably, they view it as having little to contribute to profit-making and growth, and sadly, they may be right. Moreover, as accreditation becomes commonplace, even mandatory, it runs the risk of being even less helpful. To keep it meaningful, accreditors will have to keep the bar high enough so that at least some plans do not get over it.

Above all, there is that trend towards broader, looser, include-every-physician health plans. How does a purchaser compare these kinds of "plans"? Can such plans, barely organizations of any kind, really be said to perform at all? Ironically, it seems the public demand for choice of physician may be rendering choice based on health plan quality less meaningful. If many health plans, because they include virtually all providers, end up as little more than sales organizations for providers, attempting to draw meaningful comparisons among them will be an exercise in futility. Thus, just as the science of measuring the quality of plans is improving, it may become obsolete. The task of measurement may shift to the level of provider. But at that level, obtaining accurate measurements and comparisons may prove an even more daunting task.

Overall, then, competition based on quality has a long way to go. As one typical analysis concluded, "Despite all of the attention to quality data, only a handful of purchasers are using this information to make health plan selections." Even in those markets with mature HMOs, competition having to do with quality remains based on what these researchers call the "competitive frontier" (Lipson and De Sa, 1996).

Selling Quality and Surviving Success

Unfortunately, even proving better quality may entail no guarantee that you can sell it. Quality might cost more, but employers may not be willing to pay more. Quality might be generated by creating a more integrated, tightly knit system, but until you have the reputation of the Mayo Clinic, the public may be wary of it and want more choice of physician. The goals of raising quality and offering choice, in short, conflict. Thus, between the proof of better quality and the sale of better quality may lie a sizable layer of uncertainty. Moreover, even if and when quality takes an equal place relative to price in the value equation, being the best may be fraught with risks. Here, again, we see how different health care is from other markets.

Let us consider the case of the DC-IPA (once headed by author Berenson), which contracted with a local Washington, DC HMO. Comprised of many internal medicine subspecialists, the IPA listed them as primary care gatekeepers, as well as specialists. Thus, for example, a hematologist was listed as a primary care physician, permitting patients with sickle cell disease to have a specialist in blood disorders as their primary care physician.

To network organizers it seemed like both good medical and consumer-friendly policy. But very quickly, many of the physician's sickle cell patients, who had once been enrolled in a variety of plans, began enrolling in the D.C. IPA. In that plan, after all, they would have direct access to the specialist they knew and wanted to see. To get to that specialist in other plans, they might have to go through a gatekeeper or, worse still, might not be allowed to see the specialist at all.

As a result, the D.C. IPA attracted a disproportionate share of high cost cases. The good medical, consumer-friendly practice was a poor insurance strategy and a recipe for generating losses. Reluctantly, the IPA had to ask their specialists to drop off the primary care physician list.

The lesson is painfully clear. In the insurance marketplace, avoiding high-risk enrollees pays, while attracting them costs. Plans cannot avoid these realities or the imperatives they impose. As one researcher lamented, when 30 percent of plan resources are spent on 2 percent of plan enrollees, it makes "economic sense to reduce quality just enough so that those top two per cent of members are encouraged to leave the plan" (Luft, 1997).

The problem can be seen with particular force in a review of Medicare costs. In 1996, Medicare spent almost $6,000 per beneficiary. But spending on the 10 percent of Medicare enrollees with the highest costs was almost $37,000 per beneficiary. Spending on the next most costly 10 percent was about $7,500 per beneficiary. By contrast, spending on the 70 percent with the lowest cost ranged from $0 to about $1,000 per beneficiary (Davis, 1997). Again, the lesson is clear. Health plans that attract disproportionate numbers of the highest cost enrollees will suffer. The costs they encounter will rise sharply; the payment they get from Medicare will not.

The same is true of delivery systems or providers that receive capitated payments from plans. The medical group that wins a reputation for high-quality care in treating any serious acute or chronic illness can expect to attract higher numbers of high-cost individuals. But the plan will generally pay them no more than other groups attracting more healthy populations.

This explains why many marketing strategists will advise most plans to project a reputation for good quality—but not too good. It is also why a health plan CEO decided not to offer a first-rate cancer center unless several competitors had already done it. The goal of improving quality was attractive; the likely effects of attracting more enrollees with cancer was not (Etheredge, 1997). And for the same set of reasons, you won't see an ad like this one: "Have cancer, diabetes, heart disease? Call us, we want you. Get Well health plan. Call 1-800 get well" (see figure, p. 158). A managed care plan taking this noble tack will not likely be doing it in five years. It is more likely to be in Chapter Eleven bankruptcy proceedings.

The solution to the problem seems obvious enough. Payments to plans and providers need to be "risk adjusted," based on the health status of the particular population enrolled or serviced. Thus, if a large employer or government program offered six plans, and one or two drew a higher percentage of higher cost individuals, payments to those plans would be increased. Concurrently, payments to those attracting a lower risk population would be decreased. With an appropriate risk-adjustment mechanism in place, plans and providers would be much less concerned about attracting higher cost individuals. Theoretically, at least, such enrollees might even be attractive to a plan, especially one that had learned how to care for them in the most cost-effective manner.

Unfortunately, nowhere else is the phrase "the devil is in the details" more telling. Techniques of risk adjustment are still

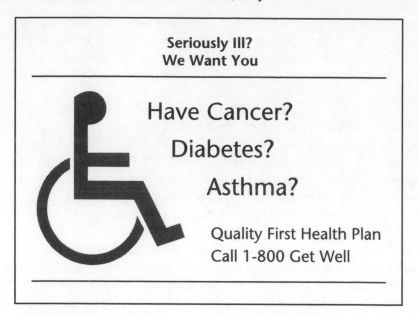

in the evolutionary stage. Only a handful of large employers, purchasing cooperatives, and state Medicaid programs are experimenting with them, and there is nothing close to a consensus on the most appropriate or fairest risk-adjustment tools. But without the capacity to adjust payments for risk, reputations for quality improvement may remain costly exercises, and incentives to develop and demonstrate higher quality may be undermined.

SUMMARY

The failure of managed care to achieve its potential to raise quality may have many causes, but a few stand out. Employers, the main purchasers of health care, focus first on price. Even if they search for value, it remains easier to do so by lowering price than by raising quality. A public demanding security in managed care defines security largely in terms of choice of physician. To date, plans have been able to provide that choice while still keeping price down. But the demand for broad choice may conflict with the requirements of higher quality, moving us back toward the old system rather than toward more integrated, coordinated systems of care. The ability to measure quality is improving, but it is still limited. Finally, proving better quality is difficult and might be costly as well.

We can blame these realities on managed care or on bottom-line-driven Wall Street forces. We can even pass all kinds of laws to attempt to force managed care organizations to change their ways. But perhaps the problem is that, in very large part, managed care is actually providing what purchasers and consumers want: lower price and choice of physician. In spite of all the talk and obvious interest of consumers in "quality," managed care organizations have not been under great pressure to produce it. Indeed, today's marketplace can actually produce reasons not to do so. This does not, however, absolve these plans of the responsibility to promote quality. But like most sellers in most markets, they will ultimately produce what is demanded of them.

We have endeavored to explore why the current marketplace is not demanding improved quality. It is now time to consider what we might do about it.

*They Can't
Take that
Away from
Me*

CONSUMER PROTECTION: TWO APPROACHES

There are two fundamentally different approaches to helping consumers get what they need and want. They are not incompatible, and many advocates of one will support elements of the other. But they stem from different views as to the nature of consumer protection and power.

The first is more traditional and is associated more with "protection" narrowly defined. It emphasizes specific definitions of consumer rights, the prevention of wrong-doing, the punishment of those doing wrong, and processes by which the wrong-doing can be corrected. As a result, it is based on government rules defining consumer rights, business obligations, and a series of dos and don'ts to which businesses must adhere. In most cases, the focus is on protection of individuals, especially those who may be more vulnerable—the elderly, the poor, the disabled, etc. In almost all instances this form of consumer protection must be imposed and enforced by government.

Consumer protection of this type may be viewed as protection of the floor. It does not attempt to define a gold standard or to enable consumers to do so on their own. Its main purposes are to protect basic needs, to make sure people do not get hurt, and to make certain that businesses live up to defined obligations and responsibilities. In a sense, it demands that all who wish to service consumers achieve and maintain a minimal standard of behavior, service, and quality.

Most of the goals of managed care regulation today, including those expressed in the current consumer backlash agenda, are of this nature. The goal of such regulation is to protect individuals from incentives inherent in managed care—specifically the incentive to skimp on care—and from inappropriate actions of managed care organizations.

The second strategy focuses less on individuals and government protection and more on the potential impact of actions taken by large numbers of consumers in the marketplace. Its goal is to serve consumers less by protecting them from wrongdoing than by empowering them in the marketplace and enabling them to make those serving them serve them better. Its tools are disclosure, information, broad-based consumer education, and more market leverage for consumers. Proponents of such a strategy would not object to fining an insurance company for harming a subscriber and forcing them to right the wrong. But they would see more protection in the public dissemination of information about the wrong-doing, which might, in turn, result in the offending company's losing customers. The insurance company that loses 10,000 enrollees, it is assumed, will quickly become a better actor in the market. To employ an old sports analogy, this strategy assumes that the best defense is a good offense.

Without question, the first strategy—the "require, investigate, and punish" approach—is critical in insurance in general, and in managed care in particular. Individuals can lose too much. The incentives to underserve can be too strong. Whatever reservations we have expressed regarding much of the anti-managed care legislation emerging in state legislatures, there should be no denying that managed care will demand more, not less, government oversight and that effective oversight includes the willingness and capacity to enforce consumer-protection rules. All of this will be especially true in the case of more vulnerable populations.

But given that the greatest failure of managed care is its inability to raise quality for all, we believe that the second, more market-oriented strategy needs more emphasis. Greater regulatory demands and more effective government oversight, however necessary, will not make managed care achieve its potential. Indeed, some elements of the current consumer-protection agenda might actually undermine the goal of improved quality for all.

In the end, consumer power may be much the same as political power, which is more the power to persuade than the authority to compel. Authority, after all, goes only so far. It is inflexible and must be defined over and over again for each special instance. In a democracy at least, the power of authority is limited and more a last resort than an everyday exercise. A governor may use it to enforce a law, but she will need some other source of power to convince legislators to pass a law.

The power to persuade, by contrast, is flexible, general, and less limited. It entails the power to get others to do things because they need or want to, not just because they have to. It can be applied to many more circumstances than those involving specific rules and regulations, and it can produce leverage in relationships with those over whom one has no formal authority (Neustadt, 1960).

The lesson for consumer protection should be evident. If consumers want the more limited power of authority—i.e., if they want to shore up the managed care floor—they need to seek more and stronger regulation-based protection. But if they want the power to persuade—i.e., if they want to raise the managed care ceiling—they need to focus more attention and energy on strengthening their leverage in the marketplace.

In this chapter, we will look at what we believe are appropriate and inappropriate steps government might take to protect the managed care floor. In Chapter 10, we will explore more market-oriented approaches to raising the managed care ceiling.

APPROACHES TO PROTECTING THE FLOOR: SOME WISE, SOME NOT

Most states already have an extensive managed care regulatory framework in place. The frameworks generally begin with a series of rules specifying what health plans must do to gain and maintain a business license, beginning with requirements that plans have the financial capacity to pay claims, including those that may be large and unexpected. To varying degrees, states also specify health-plan grievance protections, marketing and enrollment procedures, data-collection and disclosure requirements, quality monitoring, and utilization review procedures. Even before the recent managed care backlash, every state required HMOs to have a formal channel for consumer grievances. Forty-nine states required that HMOs notify enrollees that those avenues for appeal exist; thirty states even spelled out the process in some detail.

But the strength of these regulatory frameworks has varied substantially. Some states, like New York, New Jersey, Minnesota, California, Wisconsin, and Maine, now have relatively comprehensive statutes in place. In other states, regulatory frameworks have sizable gaps or make only minimal demands on managed care organizations. One late 1995 review by a California-based consumer organization concluded that "many states do not provide adequate protections for HMO enrollees. . . . In every area of consumer HMO law, we found that critical legal and regulatory issues were inadequately addressed" (Dallek, 1996). And even after the enactment of considerable backlash legislation, a 1997 review by a New York law firm characterized most states' approaches to reform as "scattershot efforts addressing politically charged, isolated issues." Laws like forty-eight-hour hospital stays for new mothers and other, isolated mandatory benefits were generally dismissed as "public policy of questionable or meager value" (Zall and others, 1997).

Enforcement of consumer protection rules is, of course, still another matter. Even the best intentioned of state regulators have found themselves hamstrung by budget cuts. In many cases, budget restrictions have hit just as the obvious needs for increased regulation of managed care have expanded. Other states just have not made adequate investments in important areas. Until recently, for example, the state of Texas, with thirty-eight licensed HMOs with over 2 million enrollees, had just one staff member in the Department of Health to investigate complaints, conduct licensing checks, and conduct on-site quality audits. Overwhelmed by the task at hand, the department hired one more individual (Azevedo, 1996).

Moreover, having a law on the books, and even an adequate personnel level, may provide no guarantee of enforcement. In California, a state with a long history of HMO activity and a generally progressive approach to consumer protection, state regulators have come under constant criticism—from government auditors, consumer groups, and the press—for weak enforcement.

Given the explosion of new forms of managed care, physician payment systems, and integrated delivery systems, it is no surprise that state regulators are continually playing catch-up with the marketplace. As one recent review published in *Medical Economics* concluded, "Few states stand out as shining examples of dependable oversight" (Azevedo, 1996).

A detailed assessment of the dozens of "consumer protection" or "anti-managed care" measures proposed or passed in recent years is far beyond our scope here. Instead, we offer a brief description of the various approaches the states and the federal government are taking, along with a quick assessment of each. Overall, we believe that policy makers and consumers must recognize the vast complexity and fluidity of the new health care marketplace and the difficulties of trying to apply fixed sets of dos and don'ts to very different circumstances. We tend to support those proposals that solidify consumer protection in areas where wrong-doing could cause the greatest harm and that improve the ability of consumers and other purchasers to evaluate and compare plans. But we are wary of proposals that unnecessarily increase costs or that may unnecessarily restrain the efforts of plans or providers to innovate and improve. Overall, our hope is to find a balance between the establishment of core, critical consumer protections and the opportunity for plans and providers to compete by improving the value of the services they offer.

Issues of Due Process

Consumer protection in managed care should begin with the right to fast-track appeals of decisions denying coverage or access to a treatment. In serious cases, patients should have access to an independent expert panel that would review the health plan's judgments based on the best clinical information available. If, for example, a plan refuses to authorize and pay for a kidney transplant—for whatever reason—the patient should be able to secure a quick review from an impartial panel of clinicians.

Reliable appeals will help ensure that health plans do not make arbitrary decisions on coverage or put financial concerns over the interests of patients. Such assurances may have value beyond their immediate purpose. Once they feel protected on this critical count, consumers may be less compelled to demand a whole host of other, less essential rights and regulations that might limit innovation or marketplace change.

Many states have already acted to secure these cornerstone protections. Others need to follow. But smart plan operators might see good reason to voluntarily adopt strong appeals processes—not to stop government from acting, but because providing these kinds of guarantees may be the best of marketing strategies.

Issues of Disclosure

Disclosure of information about plans and delivery systems plays a key role in both forms of consumer protection outlined above—those that involve specific regulatory demands, and those that rely more on impacting the marketplace. Not surprisingly, then, when it comes to disclosure, the lines between the two strategies can blur. Here we look only at those approaches to disclosure that we believe entail rights to which all consumers should be assured.

Patients and would-be subscribers should have easy access to information on such matters as plan grievance procedures, any limitations on access to in- and out-of-network physicians, and names of hospitals and other medical facilities to which plan members may be referred, or to which they could not be referred. A patient should have a right to know, for example, to what hospitals they might be sent should they require heart surgery. Basic disclosure rights should also cover payment incentives to which providers may be subjected. We may not yet have any solid research that shows how physician payment affects quality of care. But if a patient wishes to know, in general terms at least, how their physician is being paid, that information should be available to them. Additionally, to the extent that they actually limit candid discussion of treatment options and plan processes between physicians and patients, so-called "gag laws" should be barred. Plans, however, should have some rights to restrict physicians whose comments or recommendations consistently undermine patient trust in the plan. That much is common to all contractual relationships.

Disclosure rights should also be extended to critical information that might highlight poor plan performance. Such information might include: how many physicians in the plan are board certified; accreditation status of the plan; and consumer complaints filed against the plan. Of particular value may be comparative data on numbers of individuals that have disenrolled from the plan and why they did so.

Disclosure demands should also be extended to include measures of plan performance, including comparable measures of quality and consumer satisfaction. But this level of disclosure begins to reach beyond the basic disclosure rights that need to be clearly outlined in laws. We will have more to say about these approaches in Chapter 10.

Issues of Access and Quality

Today, almost all states require that HMOs have quality assurance programs. The best of them lay out processes by which plan managers (hopefully) and state regulators (if necessary) can oversee health-plan quality. These include assessment of provider credentials, physician peer review, and continuous monitoring of grievances and of care quality, especially for high-risk and chronically ill individuals. But state requirements for these programs are of very uneven quality, with many offering only limited direction as to what needs to be in the quality assurance plan (Dallek, 1996). Moreover, a strong quality assurance plan will not guarantee the delivery of quality care. Discovery of a problem is no guarantee that it will be corrected, and there is little likelihood that pressures from state regulators will force health plans to really push hard to raise quality above a minimum standard. Those kinds of pressures are far more likely to come from consumers, purchasers, and the marketplace in general (Brennan and Berwick, 1996).

But a strong quality assurance program can generate information and provide a measuring stick against which processes and goals can be judged. When combined with appropriate disclosure laws and a willingness of regulators to insist on correction of deficiencies, a strong quality assurance plan will help secure basic consumer-protection needs.

As for proposals relating to access to various providers—specialists, emergency rooms, out-of-network physicians, etc.—we find a rather mixed bag. We support, for example, a requirement that plans cover emergency room (ER) services if a "prudent layperson" goes there believing in good faith that his life or health is in imminent danger. This is good public policy. People who believe they are having a heart attack should not have to worry that they will be billed exorbitant ER fees for a false alarm.

But such rights should not be defined so broadly or inflexibly as to preclude a plan, for example, from requiring that enrollees, when possible, use ERs that are affiliated with the plan. Those ERs should have access to the plan's patient records, an enormous advantage for patients and doctors alike.

Nor should the right to coverage for an ER visit preclude plans from directing patients to urgent care centers, as opposed to high-tech, high-cost ERs. Directing a parent with a sick child running a high fever to the urgent care center might be much better for all concerned: quicker, more appropriate, and less expensive.

Many other proposals aimed at securing access to services or various providers offer much less than meets the eye. For example, measures that would guarantee consumers greater access to out-of-network or specialty physicians, or require all plans to offer a point-of-service option, may appear consumer-friendly. But they could easily raise costs and limit the capacity of managed care plans to offer different choices and trade-offs to consumers. If the Fallon Clinic in Massachusetts, a highly regarded multispecialty clinic, wishes to offer a plan that requires enrollees to see physicians associated with the clinic, why shouldn't they be allowed to do so? No employer is forced to buy it.

The most popular access proposal to date has been the so-called length-of-stay law, guaranteeing such rights as a forty-eight-hour maternity hospital stay and now a forty-eight-hour mastectomy stay. These laws may put managed care organizations on notice that excess in efforts to reduce costs can produce political reactions. But beyond their potential symbolic political value, they are clearly inappropriate. Legislators have no business making medical judgments about the specifics of appropriate care and writing them into law. Techniques, skills, treatments, and definitions of appropriate and inappropriate change too quickly. (Not too long ago, we might recall, all new mothers often stayed in the hospital for a week. Today virtually everyone would view that as grossly excessive.)

Nor is there, in almost all such cases, any data to suggest that a real problem exists. One recent study on the twenty-four-hour-stay issue found that many new mothers may have wanted more time in the hospital, but outcomes for mother and child showed no ill effects from a shorter stay (Gazmararian and others, 1997). Even if there were evidence, the appropriate point of attack would lie more in the tailored regulatory/licensing process than in the broad-brush, punish-them-all, legislative arena. Congress, for example, is certainly concerned about airline safety. But it resists writing laws about how many hours a pilot needs to rest between flights (Zall and others, 1997). Similar prudence is warranted as law makers approach hot-button issues in managed care.

Restrictions on Financial Arrangements

A number of reform proposals would limit the kinds of financial arrangements that might be negotiated between health plans and providers. Others attempt to define illegitimate levels of administrative costs or profit. These, too, we would reject.

Laws, for example, that attempt to specifically limit the amount of risk a health plan can pass on to an individual physician or group through capitation would turn out, if nothing else, to be bureaucratic quagmires. There are so many different ways (withholds, bonuses, capitation for different groups of services, etc.) of putting physicians "at risk" that defining some specific standard of acceptability, let alone trying to enforce it, would prove impossible. Worse still, passing such laws in the absence of clear evidence that certain forms of risk sharing hurt quality would stifle innovation in both integration and cost control.

A much wiser course is the requirement of disclosure of capitation arrangements—although, given the complexity of arrangements, even this may prove tricky. Plans that invoke financial incentives that are unacceptably strong will face problems in the marketplace. Strengthened grievance procedures, as outlined earlier, will also help. Together, these reforms should provide a sound balance between strengthening consumer protection and allowing for the exploration of options in managed care financing. As we have argued, some of those options might offer means to higher quality.

Similarly, while proposals that would define a percent of each premium dollar that must go to direct patient care, as opposed to administration or profit (the so-called minimum-loss ratio), may seem likely to limit profiteering, such rules are easily manipulated, impose unnecessary rigidity on plan arrangements, and may have little to do with quality of care. The imposition of such formulas can produce grossly misleading sets of numbers. For example, some plans consider "quality assurance" to be a medical expense, not an administrative cost. As a result, their numbers look better, as if they are spending more on care and less on administration.

Rigid formulas can also punish plans that spend considerable "administrative" resources on physician selection and recruitment or on new information systems that improve clinical practice. Their loss-ratio numbers will look worse. Plans, on the other hand, that tolerate old-system approaches of paying too many physicians for doing more than what is necessary may have low administrative costs and better loss-ratio numbers. They may spend more on "medical care," as opposed to "administration." But they and their enrollees will get much less for their money.

If the urge to legislate in this area is too compelling to resist, disclosure might again suffice. And, in the cases of laws on both physician-plan relationships and loss ratios, giving consumers more choice of plan offers a preferred alternative. Consumers or purchasers who do not like the way a particular plan operates can ask questions, or go elsewhere.

New Delivery Systems

In Chapter 5 we described how many California HMOs work. The employer contracts with an insurer, who then contracts with a number of medical groups, usually paying them a capitation payment covering most or all medical services for a fixed population. Consumers then pick a physician and the medical group with which the physician is affiliated.

In these arrangements, the role of the insurance company is substantially diminished. The medical group selects physicians, develops its own utilization review procedures, decides who will get what services and under what conditions, and reviews patient grievances. Unlike the traditional insurance arrangement, the providers bear most or all of the "risk" for the population covered. In other words, if the patient group gets sicker than expected, the providers—not the insurer—would lose money. In such situations, the provider acts and looks increasingly like an insurer.

In different forms—and especially in integrated delivery systems—this blurring of the distinction between insurer and provider is happening in many regions. And under the Balanced Budget Act Medicare reforms enacted in 1997, it may happen even more frequently. Groups of providers—called provider-sponsored organizations (PSOs)—will be allowed to contract with the Medicare program to provide care to Medicare recipients, without the insurer acting as an intermediary.

We see considerable potential in these trends. They can encourage integration among providers and enable consumers to pick among local delivery systems. The ability to choose among local delivery systems should also advantage the consumer interested in seeking out quality.

But in terms of consumer protection, there is a risk here. To date, almost all consumer-protection legislation has focused on the regulation of insurers. Integrated delivery systems, large medical groups, multispecialty clinics, and physician-hospital organizations are largely unregulated. Individuals working in them may have to be licensed, but unless the organization seeks an insurance license, it is likely to face few if any requirements. As organizations, they are generally regulated only indirectly through the insurance system, in that insurers must make certain that the providers with whom they contract meet certain standards and abide by various requirements.

But what happens when there is no insurer in the picture, as will be the case with the new PSOs? Today, this is one of health care's hottest issues. Health plans want a "level playing field," in which any medical group or integrated health system that takes full capitation or risk is required to be licensed like any insurer. Provider groups want more leeway than that. They want the option to go directly to purchasers, and many want to assume risk and the potential for profit and autonomy it can offer. But they do not want to bear the burdens or requirements—to offer certain mandated benefits or to abide by various solvency, disclosure, or grievance procedure rules—that states place on insurers.

We favor the flexibility to explore the new relationships. But we also fear that if integrated systems, including the new breed of PSOs, function outside of consumer-protection frameworks, consumers could end up with more choices but less protection of fundamental consumer rights. Overall, we remain unconvinced that groups or providers who are, in effect, providing health insurance should be free of requirements that

---

Who Is at Risk?
(And Who Should Be Regulated?)

Provider Sponsored Organization Tasks	Insurer Tasks
• Provide all care	• Maintain license
• Utilization review and quality assurance	• Contract with buyers
• Provider selection	• Reinsurance
• Coverage decision-making	• Marketing
• Info services	• Data reporting and dissemination
• Provider payment	• Enrollment/administration
• Claims processing	• May supply capital
• Access to providers	• Actuarial services
• Global capitation	

---

insurers have to meet. If, of course, those requirements offer more burden than protection, they should be eliminated for all. But that is a separate question.

Medicaid and Medicare

Expansion of managed care to the Medicaid and Medicare populations has, overall, been more successful than many thought it would be. Marketing abuses have been less extreme than those that occurred in earlier expansions of these programs, as in California in the 1970s. Many states, such as New York, have acted to reduce abuses and the tendency of Medicaid managed care programs to become the "Medicaid mills" of the past.

But the poor and the elderly have special needs. Some confront language barriers. Many suffer from chronic illnesses. They may be less equipped to assert their rights in managed care organizations. Some may be more susceptible to salespersons who promise more than will be delivered. For these and many other reasons, history suggests the need to err on the side of too much rather than too little consumer protection.

As the rush to lower government costs moves literally tens of millions of Medicare and Medicaid recipients into managed care plans, especially HMOs, ongoing, aggressive monitoring of these transitions will be essential. In the Medicaid program, the biggest threat may lie in the lack of regulatory capacity to adequately monitor quality and service in managed care plans. Risks will be especially high as enrollment moves from primarily young and healthy women and their children, to include those with the most chronic and high-cost illnesses and disabilities. Even where state regulators wish to do it right, they lack the capacity to do so. They will need to tailor the speed of their transitions to managed care to their capacity to monitor the transition.

In the Medicare program, the 1997 reforms offer both opportunity and challenge. On paper, the new system looks like a free-market, consumer-choice dream. Medicare beneficiaries will have a wealth of choices: traditional Medicare, HMOs, PPOs, PSOs, and even private fee-for-service plans. But helping beneficiaries sift through and understand the choices poses an enormous challenge. Moreover, the incentives for delivery systems and insurers to seek out the healthy and avoid the sick remain as powerful as ever. To make the new system work, Medicare will implement risk adjustment mechanisms that are largely untested. It should also consider easing the consumer's decision-making burden and improving the consumer's capacity to choose, by invoking some degree of benefits standardization.

Provider Protections

Many of the access proposals we discussed earlier, like those guaranteeing access to out-of-network providers, have been supported and even written by medical associations seeking to undermine network approaches. Related policies are more explicitly about protecting doctors themselves from the economic forces unleashed by managed care. Among them, the most conspicuous are "any willing provider" laws that guarantee physicians' rights to participate in any health plan network so long as they abide by network rules.

For reasons we have already discussed, these policies undermine health plans' ability to control costs and select for quality. Certainly, many plans are more interested in whether physicians will accept their reduced rates than whether they might improve quality. But the appropriate fix is to identify inferior plans and allow consumers and purchasers the options to go elsewhere; it is not to make all plans look alike and to turn the better ones into mediocre ones. Networks and managed care organizations should have the right to select physicians they want and to keep out those they do not want.

Rights of physicians to stay in a network are another matter. So, too, are the rights of patients, who can suffer if their physician is dropped from a network. Indeed, many consumers sign up with a given plan *because* their physician is a participant in the plan's network. To the extent possible, their rights to continued access to a physician dropped by a network should be maintained. But as for rights of physicians, their remedy may lie in contracts with plans, not in state law. Physicians can seek contracts that offer specified protection regarding network participation.

The one area in which government may have a compelling interest here is in the protection of physicians who attract high-cost patients, either because of where they practice or because of their reputation for effective or compassionate service to those with great need. If plans feel free to drop such physicians because they raise plan costs, physicians, like insurers, will feel pressures to avoid serving the most needy. Clearly, there is no public interest in going down that road. Still, the best answer here may not be a new series of regulations, but advances in risk-adjustment methodologies, so that providers and plans with higher cost patients may be paid more.

The Employee Retirement Income Security Act

Even if state legislatures passed all the right consumer-protection laws, about half of all Americans insured through employer-sponsored plans would find the laws did not apply to them. Self-insured plans are governed by a federal law, the Employee Retirement Income Security Act of 1974, or ERISA, which is woefully weak in its consumer-protection provisions. As one review by the National Health Policy Forum concluded, "The combination of restricted federal authority, scarce resources, and ERISA's narrow judicial remedies is likely to leave people in self-insured plans without adequate means to resolve plan coverage disputes" (Butler and Polzer, 1966).

Thus, in one widely noted case, an employer operating a benefits plan under ERISA was able to rewrite its health plan to place a $5,000 cap on AIDS benefits, an adjustment that would be prohibited were employees enrolled with a state-licensed insurer (Physician Payment Review Commission, 1996). ERISA plans are also free of state requirements to offer certain benefits, such as coverage of mammograms.

Moreover, ERISA plans are often administered by insurers. As a result, many individuals in ERISA plans do not even realize they are in one, let alone what that may mean in terms of consumer protection. Stories abound in which individuals have complained to employers or administrators that they were denied a benefit (e.g., a free annual mammogram) or right (e.g., the right to an expedited hearing) granted in state law—only to find out that state law did not apply.

In ERISA plans, consumer protection is largely dependent on the willingness of the employer to deliver it. Many employers do. Some self-insured employers are among the most responsible "insurers" in the country. Many have been leaders in the effort to improve quality in health care delivery. Still, self-insured plans remain the great black hole of consumer protection.

Unfortunately, the employers that operate ERISA plans—that is, most of the Fortune 500 companies and thousands of others—vigorously oppose even modest reform. Moreover, ERISA reform constitutes a Herculean public-education challenge. To address it, consumer groups need to raise public awareness of a law about which even some health policy experts know very little. In comparison to rallying consumers around a forty-eight-hour length-of-stay law or a right to see physicians outside a network, persuading consumers to amend the ERISA "preemption" is a nightmarish task. It might be explained in a *New York Times* op-ed piece, but it will never make the news at eleven.

ERISA reform, then, should be on the front burner of the consumer-protection agenda, but, until very recently, it hasn't been. In 1997, with consumers in full throat over managed care, two researchers reported that they "couldn't identify any consumer advocacy organization focusing on ERISA health care issues" (Polzer and Butler, 1997).

The ERISA issue, of course, along with the perceived weakness of many state regulatory frameworks and the nationalization of managed care concerns, has focused attention on a broader question: What is the proper role of the federal government in supplementing and supporting what are essentially state consumer-protection responsibilities? The answer may be neither obvious nor politically achievable. Certainly, the nationalization of the debate has been valuable, forcing policy makers to focus on critical issues and concerns. In particular, as members of Congress have asserted federal authority in consumer protection, they have been forced to confront the ERISA problem: that unless they do something about ERISA, consumer-protection laws will remain ineffectual for millions. One option, strongly advocated by consumer groups, is to establish a federal floor of core consumer-protection provisions, a kind of national consumer bill of rights, with enforcement at the state level and states able to add protections on top of it.

But even if action at the federal level might fill some gaps and offer symbolic value, the vast majority of consumer-protection capacity—in legislation and certainly enforcement—is going to, and should, remain with the states. In most respects, the states win the jurisdictional argument hands down. They can more easily adjust rules and regulations to different marketplaces. They can be more flexible in allowing for experimentation and innovation in regulatory approaches. Above all, states have a capacity to enforce consumer protection that the federal government does not have. There is no federal equivalent to a state department of insurance, and there won't be.

To the extent, then, that consumer advocates wish to strengthen consumer protection, they may want to make a case at the federal level. But they will need to pass laws and demand enforcement at the state level.

Consumer Protection: Regulatory and Market-Based Power

When Harry Christie of California sought to have a specialist at Stanford Medical Center University operate on his daughter for a rare form of cancer, his HMO, Take Care, refused to pay. They wanted him to use a different surgeon at the same hospital who had never performed the required surgery on children. Christie ended up paying for the surgeon of his choice; using the Take Care grievance process would have taken too long. But Take Care refused to reimburse him for the surgeon's fees or even for the $47,000 in hospital costs that presumably would have had to be paid even if the surgeon Take Care recommended had been used. Several months of appeals through the Take Care grievance processes produced no relief. Only when Christie pursued the matter through arbitration was it determined that Take Care owed Christie for both the surgeon and hospital fees. California regulators would eventually fine Take Care $500,000 for endangering the patient's life and violating quality standards (Rodwin, 1996).

The story offers a compelling example of the need for strong consumer-protection measures in managed care relationships.

If we look below the surface, though, we may also see the limits of such protection. For example, we have argued that the institution of stronger grievance procedures may be the single most important specific protection that consumers might seek today. But the fact is that such procedures, even when they exist and include appeals to outside powers, are not used very much (Iglehart, 1997). They can be complex. They can take time to pursue and time to resolve. And using them may be intimidating for many consumers, especially when they are "locked in" to the system they are challenging. It's one thing to complain about Sears when you can buy tires at fifteen other stores. It's another thing to complain—especially if you are ill and vulnerable—about a physician or an HMO when you can't leave your insurance plan for a year or when your employer offers no other option.

Moreover, viewing the problem from a broader public interest perspective, positive outcomes of grievance procedures—unlike the Take Care case cited above—may have only minimal impact. They will benefit the individual consumer involved, but they will not necessarily force the managed care organization to change its ways. The next consumer may have to fight the issue all over again.

Thus, even the most critical of regulatory consumer-protection elements has big limitations. This leads us back to the core reality, that the biggest gains in consumer protection, broadly defined, are likely to come in the form of market-based strategies. It is to those options that we now turn.

10
Thirteen Steps to Raising Quality in Managed Care

With a Little Help from My Friends

Managed care's major failure has not been the harm it may have caused the few, but its lackluster performance in improving quality for the many. As a result, an agenda focused on improving managed care must reach beyond the prevention of wrong-doing to individuals, to means by which managed care organizations can be encouraged to raise the quality of care for all. It must be an agenda not of reaction, but of opportunity.

Outlined below is one such agenda. It assumes that consumers will need more than additional legal protections or legislated lists of services that managed care plans must offer. They will need the market power to force managed care plans to deliver the highest quality at the lowest possible price. History shows us that companies are less likely to get serious about quality when it is dictated by a government rule than when their survival in the marketplace demands it.

Our agenda focuses on the consumer because we believe the consumer should be in the health care driver's seat. But employers, providers, and policy makers also have major roles to play and tools with which to pressure managed care to do better.

1. FROM EMPLOYER TO EMPLOYEE CHOICE

While fee-for-service health plans were all pretty much the same, today's managed health plans can be very different from one another. They offer not only a variety of quality and price, but different trade-offs between such factors as cost, access, and choice. Some plans are simply better than others. Especially for people who have unique or substantial health care needs, being a member of one plan or another can make a major difference.

For these and many other reasons, employees should be choosing their own health plans. Employers can pay for health care, as they have in the past. They can assist their workers in buying insurance by providing good information about the strengths and weaknesses of the plans in the community. But the choice itself should shift from employer to employee. Perhaps no other change in our health care system would do more to reward quality and value in managed care.

The ripple effects of such a change would be substantial. Employee choice will eliminate the confusion as to who is the health plan's number-one customer. Today, an HMO has more reason to lavish attention on the human resources managers of major corporations than on the employees who will be its patients. Employee choice will also give the health care consumer the ultimate leverage possessed by consumers in most marketplaces: the ability to leave. It will increase the probability that changing jobs will not mean changing plans or providers. It will also mean that physicians will not have to join all plans to maintain relationships with loyal patients. Indeed, employee choice of plan will do much more to improve the power balance between plans and physicians than anti-competitive, "any willing provider" type legislation that physicians misguidedly endorse. Most important, it will increase the likelihood that at least some plans will make new and greater efforts to improve and market quality.

Employee choice may also lead health plans to differentiate themselves more aggressively in the eyes of consumers. Today's focus on the employer as purchaser forces plans to employ a "lowest common denominator" approach to marketing. The employer is interested in offering, at most, a few plans that will be acceptable to the majority of employees. Plans respond by offering options geared to appeal to all. As a result, health plans begin to look the same. In today's marketplace, that tends to mean offering broader choice of physician. Offering less choice might be appealing to some, but unappealing to too many. When so many employers are purchasing just one plan, being a bit different is too risky an option.

Some might suggest that employers would make better choices because they know more about value-based purchasing than their employees. Where employers believe that is true, we suggest that they help their employees to make smart decisions. But the vast majority of employers know little or nothing about purchasing health care. Moreover, we find this "employer knows best" view unacceptably paternalistic. Employers pay employees for doing a job; they are not their guardians. They make workplace but not lifestyle decisions for their employees.

Skeptics might also note that research to date suggests that the sophistication level of individuals in choosing health care plans is modest at best. This, of course, is true. But the realities of today need not be, and would not be, the realities of tomorrow. The limited capacity of consumers to choose health plans may simply reflect their lack of experience in doing it and the absence of intermediaries around to help them do it. Recall that about 50 percent of employees have no choice of plan. They have bought many more TVs, cars, appliances, and car insurance policies than health plans. They have had to choose plumbers, tax accountants, stock brokers, and maybe even lawyers. But many have never had to choose a health plan.

In making many of these choices, consumers have all kinds of helpers. A small industry exists, for example, to assist consumers in buying cars. The average car buyer may test drive five cars, ask ten friends about their cars, review two car-buying guides (one of them on the Internet), and visit five different showrooms. But how much time have most of us spent assessing health plans?

To imagine the capacity of individual consumers to make health plan choices, we need to look ahead five or ten years and envision a system in which most Americans choose their own plans and have done so four or five times. *Consumer Reports* and other such intermediaries—for-profit and not-for-profit—will be offering periodic regional reports on provider performance, health plan quality, and consumer satisfaction. Governments, employers, and purchasing coalitions will be collecting and disseminating all kinds of standardized information about plans and providers.

"Eventually," as one analyst puts it, "the curtain of ignorance (in choosing health plans) will lift" (Kerr, 1997). In the end, there is no reason consumers should not begin to approach the same level of competency in choosing health plans as they assert in choosing cars, universities, stereo equipment, department stores, lawyers, or homes. Some of these, we should recognize, are very difficult choices.

2. EXPANDING CONSUMER CHOICE TO DELIVERY SYSTEMS, NOT JUST INSURERS

The Medicare modifications enacted by Congress in 1997 open the door to direct contracting between the Medicare program and groups of providers, called provider service organizations (PSOs). These reforms acknowledged a trend already evident in some markets: organizations of physicians, and sometimes physicians and hospitals, have been seeking to bypass insurers and contract directly with employers. In the new Medicare model, individuals will have a plethora of choices, including HMOs, traditional Medicare, and the new PSO.

Employers, providers, and consumers all have good reasons to encourage and explore this new avenue of health care purchasing. Instead of choosing among Aetna, Prudential, and Blue Cross, the consumer might choose among a large local medical group, a system organized by a local Catholic hospital, another centered around the local university medical center, and even many traditional HMOs like Kaiser.

This kind of delivery-system choice might promote competition on quality, as it may be easier for consumers to judge the quality of a local delivery system than that of a national insurer. Delivery-system choice might also encourage integration and coordination among providers; achieving higher levels of both would be critical for providers sharing risk and competing as a system.

How we broaden choice to include delivery systems is another matter. The Medicare approach, by which individuals choose among insurers *and* delivery systems, is one model. California, where insurers offer consumers a long list of group-affiliated primary care physicians, is another. A coalition of large self-insured employers in Minnesota offers still another variation on the same theme. The coalition pays one HMO an administrative fee. That HMO then manages a menu of competing medical groups, who are responsible for providing a comprehensive benefits package. Then employees choose among the medical groups, not insurers.

In some forms, the choose-a-delivery-system approach is fraught with regulatory complexities. These will, no doubt, be a source of great revenue to health care lawyers across the country. As noted in Chapter 9, purchasers and policy makers will need to make certain that critical consumer-protection measures that now affect licensed insurers do not fall away as control shifts from insurers to providers. Selection of delivery systems will also require that the current focus on comparing the performance of health plans be extended to the performance of providers—an even more complex task.

Still, consumer leaders, unions, and employee groups interested in promoting competition on quality should be studying these kinds of options. Legal complexities do not have to stand in the way.

3. ENHANCING THE POWER OF THE PURCHASER

The California Health Insurance Purchasing Cooperative (HIPC), established by government, is a purchasing coalition serving over 7,000 small firms with about 135,000 employees and dependents. It is open to all companies with 2 to 50 employees. All groups pay the same rates, adjusted only for the region and for the age and sex of the employees and their dependents. The HIPC selects and offers a wide choice of plans and types of plans, including POS, PPO and HMO plans. Consumers choose their own plans. Benefits are largely standardized, so that consumers can more easily compare plans on price and quality. The HIPC negotiates with plans over rates and distributes information about plan performance, consumer satisfaction, and other factors. It has even begun a unique effort to implement a risk-adjustment strategy in which plans that enroll higher cost individuals get paid more.

Some large employers, either on their own or in coalition with others, invoke similar purchasing strategies. But small employers cannot do these things alone. They have virtually no expertise or market clout. And their administrative costs are much too high to even consider offering a choice of plans. They need help, and the purchasing coalition may be the best way to get it.

Through coalitions, the small and even mid-sized employer can reap the advantages of larger purchasers: lower administrative costs, more bargaining clout with plans, investment in purchasing expertise, increased dissemination of information about plan choices, and an ability to put purchasing choices in the hands of employees rather than employers.

Large companies can also benefit from the coalition approach. They like to think that having 5,000–10,000 employees produces market leverage. But a purchasing coalition controlling tens of thousands of "covered lives" can generate a different perspective. And a coalition like that of California state and local government purchasers, with over a million "covered lives," can move markets.

Until recently, such leverage had generally been used only to achieve lower prices. But as their levels of sophistication and expertise have grown, some large purchasers or coalitions have begun using their leverage to demand quality-related change as well. Many now collect and disseminate data comparing plans, and at least one now disseminates information on local medical groups as well (*Pacific Currents*, 1997). Some stipulate that they will only offer accredited plans. The Pacific Business Group on Health has stolen a page from the HMO payment book in purchasing insurance for large California employers and actually withholds modest percentages of premiums until contracted plans improve on specified quality measures. If immunization rates do not increase within the next six months, they pay 2 percent less.

Unfortunately, where the need is greatest—the small-group market—the difficulties of invoking the coalition strategy have proven considerable. Small-group purchasing coalitions, expected by many to flourish, have encountered all kinds of roadblocks. Employers are focused on producing and marketing widgets, not buying health care. Some may be reluctant to enter arrangements that employees may like too much and begin to view as a right. Insurance brokers, whose role the coalition can easily undermine, tend to view them with fear and loathing. Insurers also have little use for them, perhaps recognizing their potential to increase the demands and sophistication of purchasers.

Given these obstacles, and the advantages of the coalition approach for consumers in particular, the coalition deserves a helping hand from public policy makers. Start-up grants could be offered. So, too, could expertise—especially on such complex matters as risk-adjustment methodologies. Government mailers to small employers could include information about coalition options. Government purchasers could open up their own purchasing pools—including the 19-million-member Federal Employee Health Benefits Program—to small employers, enabling the latter to "buy in" to the services, expertise, and leverage of the public purchaser. Finally, some rules for small-group coalitions would be required, lest coalitions begin to compete like insurers have competed—on the basis of who is best at avoiding high-risk enrollees.

The coalition movement also could use help from consumer groups. Given their compelling potential, it is striking that consumers and consumer organizations are doing little to press for the wider adoption of coalitions, or even for the institution of greater consumer choice of plan. Perhaps it is because they are investing so much of their limited political energy in protecting the managed care floor. In fact, as the coalition example suggests, the goal of improving quality in managed care plans might be advanced considerably if consumers were to place less emphasis on regulation-based protection and more on strengthening their own market power. Such efforts might focus on greater education of consumers about choices available to them; increased pressures on employers to offer employees choice or to join or form purchasing coalitions; and lobbying efforts directed at getting state and federal governments to facilitate the establishment of purchasing coalitions, especially in the small-employer marketplace. Some of these market-based efforts to improve quality might even encounter less opposition than regulatory approaches, which inevitably raise red flags about too much government.

4. TOWARD MORE COST-CONSCIOUS CONSUMERS

The Federal Employee Health Benefits Plan is often cited as a model purchaser, but the purchasing strategy it employs has at least one flaw. Because the government pays about 75 percent of the costs of any plan chosen, it lays out more money when employees choose higher cost plans. In this respect, it makes higher cost plans a better deal.

Let us contrast this with an approach in which the employer makes a fixed contribution, say $2,000 for an individual employee's health benefits. (Contributions for employees with dependents would be higher.) The $2,000 might pay 80 percent or even 100 percent of the lowest cost plan available to the employee. The employee then chooses from a menu of plans, some of which may cost more than $2,000 per year. If the employee chooses one of those more expensive plans, he pays the full difference between the $2,000 and the cost of the plan he chooses. This contribution strategy raises the cost-consciousness of employees, requiring those who choose a higher cost plan to see and pay the full, higher cost of the plan.

Whether the higher cost plan is worth the price is up to the individual. But the contribution strategy helps the employee to see and evaluate health care trade-offs. Not only does the employee who wants a more expensive plan pay more, but, just as important, the employee who chooses a lower cost plan pays less. The result can be employees and health care purchasers with a better understanding of value.

Employer Contribution Methods and Cost Conscious Employee Choice of Plan

Employer pays 100% of premium of any plan chosen	Employer pays a percent of premium of any plan chosen	Employer pays a fixed dollar amount applied to any plan chosen	Employer pays all or a portion of lowest cost plan only
Least incentive for cost conscious choice ———————————————————➤			Greatest incentive for cost conscious choice

---

This practice need not, we should emphasize, reduce the overall contribution of the employer. The fixed contribution could be 100 percent of a relatively high-cost, comprehensive benefits plan. The critical factor is that employees who want still more should pay the full extra cost of more. Moreover, as the economist will advise us, if the employer does pay less overall, the employees will ultimately get the employer's savings in the form of higher wages or other benefits.

Consumer understanding of health care cost trade-offs would also be reinforced by placing a limit on the tax deductibility of health benefits. Exempting the cost of a standard benefits package (e.g., $1,500-$2,000 for an individual) from taxes makes sense. But as we described in Chapter 1, granting tax exemptions for more lavish benefits packages or plans that charge more than necessary to deliver a standard, comprehensive benefits package sends all the wrong signals. Worse still, current tax policy is highly regressive. The people with the biggest and most expensive benefits packages, generally the wealthier among us, get the biggest tax deductions in dollars (e.g., $2,500 vs. $2,000), and because they are in higher tax brackets (e.g., 28 percent vs. 15 percent), their higher deduction goes further. At the other end of the spectrum, the low-wage employee with no health insurance gets no tax break at all.

Unfortunately, changing tax policy here has been a political nonstarter. Democrats might see the change as progressive, especially if the deduction were replaced by a credit. But unions, many of which have negotiated sizable benefits packages, are strongly opposed. Republicans sometimes see the economic logic of improving consumer cost-consciousness and of reducing what is, in effect, a sizable government-spending program. But eliminating or reducing the deduction would be branded by opponents as a "tax increase." A change in this policy, then, may have to await a moment of bipartisan vision or political change of heart.

5. GETTING SOPHISTICATED: THE SUBTLER HEALTH CARE TRADE-OFFS

Consumer understanding of health care trade-offs may start with costs, but must get beyond them. Many other, much subtler trade-offs need to be faced. The most critical of these involve integration, quality, and choice. As we have argued, systems that are more highly integrated—including more physician attachment to the system, more coordination of care, better information systems, more use of protocols and guidelines, etc.—have greater potential for delivering higher quality care. But integrated systems offer less choice of physician. Thus, it will be hard to find integration, quality, and wide choice under one health care tent. To a point at least, more integration and higher quality may be more compatible with less, not more, choice.

Today, choice is winning the competition. Enrollment growth has been far more dramatic among plans offering more choice. Many more integrated plans have been experiencing much more modest growth.

Until more integrated managed care systems do a better job of proving their value, most consumers will continue to choose choice over integration. But the tendency to undermine integration in the pursuit of choice, as seen in some legislative proposals today, must be resisted. The far more appropriate response would be to move toward employee choice of plan, as previously explained. If employees were free to choose their own plans, they could choose plans with which their personal physician was associated. They might then be less concerned about physician choice *within* a plan. Under this circumstance, the potential conflict between choice of physician and plan integration would be reduced. Choice and quality could go forward, hand in hand.

6. IMPROVING THE ABILITY TO CHOOSE: THE INFORMATION REVOLUTION, PART ONE

Information will be the lifeblood of the new health care system.

Fortunately, a small information revolution is already under way. The quantity of information available on performance of health plans, consumer satisfaction in health plans, accreditation status of health plans, and even the internal decision-making processes and quality of care delivered by health plans is growing in multiples. Digital Equipment Corporation, for example, informs employees about the percentage of primary care physicians who are board certified and even about the percentage of phone calls to the plan that are answered within twenty seconds. California State employees are told how many of their fellow employees switched from one plan to another and why (Moskowitz, 1997). The recent release by the NCQA of its Quality Compass 1997 (described in Chapter 7) is unprecedented in scope and detail, and much of it can be found on the Internet. And overall, the information available on health plan performance "report cards" today is far richer and more usable than anything available just a few years ago (see, for example, the Performance Reports on the various California plans, pages 190–191).

Consumer, rather than employer, choice of plans would encourage this revolution, creating a far larger market for such information, and offering rich opportunities for intermediaries, like new publications, web sites, or consumer groups, that might produce and disseminate more consumer-oriented information.

Performance Reports Coming of Age
Comparing California Plans 1996

California Health Plans	Cervical Cancer Screening	Childhood Immuni- zation	Diabetic Retinal Exam
Aetna Health Plans of CA-North	73	71 ▲	48 ▲
Aetna Health Plans of CA-San Diego	76 ▲	73 ▲	38
Aetna Health Plans of CA-South	59 ▼	59	36
Blue Cross/California Care	69	58	29 ▼
Blue Shield of California	63	58	29 ▼
CareAmerica	55 ▼	54 ▼	27 ▼
CIGNA HealthCare of Northern CA	67	72 ▲	31 ▼
CIGNA HealthCare of San Diego	64	58	29 ▼
CIGNA HealthCare of Southern CA	63	52 ▼	30 ▼
FHP/TakeCare	63	62	42
Foundation Health	59 ▼	50 ▼	26 ▼
Health Net	75 ▲	61	42
Health Plan of the Redwoods	82 ▲	67 ▲	43 ▲
Kaiser Permanente of Northern CA	78 ▲	78 ▲	54 ▲
Kaiser Permanente of Southern CA	70	64	58 ▲
Lifeguard	75 ▲	67 ▲	41
Maxicare	58 ▼	61	
National Health Plan	62 ▼	49 ▼	27 ▼
Omni Healthcare	69	59	33
PacificCare of California	75 ▲	63	34
Prudential HealthCare HMO	61 ▼	55 ▼	38
United HealthCare	66	63	34
Average of All Plans Surveyed	67	62	37

Key to Performance Strata
  00 ▲ = above average
  00   = average
  00 ▼ = below average

Performance Reports Coming of Age
(continued)

California Health Plans	Breast Cancer Screening	Prenatal Care	Advise to Quit Smoking †
Aetna Health Plans of CA-North	75 ▲	94 ▲	64
Aetna Health Plans of CA-San Diego	71	91 ▲	64
Aetna Health Plans of CA-South	64	80	60
Blue Cross/California Care	64	78	70
Blue Shield of California	71	77	71
CareAmerica	60 ▼	70 ▼	58
CIGNA HealthCare of Northern CA	71	80	64
CIGNA HealthCare of San Diego	67	94 ▲	67
CIGNA HealthCare of Southern CA	65	68 ▼	57
FHP/TakeCare	67	88 ▲	60
Foundation Health	63 ▼	57 ▼	59
Health Net	70	87 ▲	52
Health Plan of the Redwoods	73 ▲	96 ▲	66
Kaiser Permanente of Northern CA	75 ▲	89 ▲	63
Kaiser Permanente of Southern CA	77 ▲	90 ▲	62
Lifeguard	77 ▲	94 ▲	70
Maxicare	58 ▼	74 ▼	52
National Health Plan	69	88 ▲	
Omni Healthcare	77 ▲	72 ▼	67
PacificCare of California	72	90 ▲	56
Prudential HealthCare HMO	64	68 ▼	65
United HealthCare	62 ▼	79	
Average of All Plans Surveyed	69	82	62

Key to Performance Strata
  00 ▲ = above average
  00   = average
  00 ▼ = below average

† Performance strata (above average, average, and below average) could not be determined for this measure because of small sample sizes.

Source: Adapted from California Cooperative Health Care Reporting Initiative.

So, too, might the growth of purchasing coalitions. Among other things, the formation of coalitions would spur the development of a larger pool of expert purchasers. Whether they used that expertise to select plans from which coalition members would then choose, to demand improvement from participating plans, or to inform consumers about the plans offered, the emergence of a professional and active class of experts in health care purchasing would be of enormous value.

Pursuit of the information revolution will require some government direction. If, for example, other states or the federal government wish to duplicate New York State's program on monitoring and comparing outcomes in open heart surgery, government action will be required—to compel providers and hospitals to produce the results, to determine the standardized format in which the results are to be collected, and to assure that the data is accurate. In general, standardization offers two obvious advantages: it eases the burden on providers and plans who need to respond to one request rather than many, and it enhances the ability of all to compare the information generated. Today, the debate on standardization and who should do it—at least within health policy circles—is pretty hot. But it will be difficult to move toward standardization without some government involvement.

Finally, for those concerned about the lack of quantifiable information available on health-plan quality, or about that dearth of information limiting the ability of consumers to choose their own plans, we suggest that the bar and expectations not be set too high. Comparing managed care organizations on objective quantifiable criteria is a noble goal, but what other complex economic organizations can we compare in this way? Airlines? Universities? Department stores? Supermarkets? In each case, one can choose a few criteria that can be measured or standardized. But, in the end, we consult experts (who may differ), listen to friends and family, review our own experiences, apply our own set of values, and then make what are largely personal, subjective choices. That health care purchasing might not be much different should hardly alarm us.

7. IMPROVING CLINICAL PERFORMANCE:
THE INFORMATION REVOLUTION, PART TWO

A revolution is also taking place in the generation of information on what works and does not work in health care delivery. The initial 1970s studies on practice variations are now part of a veritable "atlas" of such data, and the quality and quantity of such information will continue to improve and expand. Here, too, a government role is essential. Sophisticated research on clinical outcomes is expensive. Health plans or delivery systems are not likely to undertake major efforts on their own. Even when they do, they have an interest in keeping what they learn proprietary. Yet, keeping clinical advances and knowledge private does not serve public interests. (It may even violate medical ethics.)

Consequently, if the public values such research—and we should—government is going to have to pay for it. And since the private sector is not likely to disseminate research findings, government will need to assume responsibility for this function as well. Alternatively, of course, government could require that all plans contribute a small fraction of premiums collected to fund and disseminate research. But, either way, government has to see that it happens.

8. FROM OPPOSITION TO LEADERSHIP:
THE ROLE OF PHYSICIANS

Throughout the managed care revolution, most physicians and their organizations have fought a defensive battle. They have objected to the tools, the restraints, the pressures to reduce costs, and the loss of physician autonomy that managed care arrangements impose. They have fought with public relations efforts, by backing legislation that would guarantee them more rights vis-à-vis managed care plans, and with efforts to undermine public confidence in the new system.

In doing so, doctors have sometimes muddied the distinction between patients' interests and their own. Over time, this will not serve them well. If each time physicians are seen as "patient advocates" they are also perceived as advocating policies that benefit themselves, leadership opportunities and public confidence will be hard to come by.

Admittedly, the new system poses stiff challenges for physicians, especially those intent on maintaining a commitment to a patient-first ethic. Under fee-for-service, there was little conflict for an ethical physician. Putting the patient first in a capitated payment system, however, might affect the physician's income; it could even risk alienating health plans upon which physicians must rely for business.

But physicians need to start directing managed care rather than just opposing it. Their constructive criticism and efforts to push the new system toward improved quality are sorely needed and could prove an enormous asset to consumers. Physicians need to point out where managed care strategies pose dangers for consumers. They need to take the lead in developing tools and methods that will better enable all concerned to compare plans and providers on quality-related measures, including outcomes of care. Doctors could conduct and publish their own surveys on health-plan quality. And most important, they need to blow the whistle on plans that impose policies that undermine quality of care or consumer rights, a duty which includes their willingness to walk away from bad plans. (Again, consumer choice would help here. Patients could follow their physicians, and leaving a plan would not necessarily mean losing patients enrolled in the plan.)

Recently, some physicians have seemed more amenable to change and thereby have tried to influence the future of managed care. For example, a 1997 *Wall Street Journal* article reported on a pair of cardiologists in Minneapolis who were chafing under an HMO's rules regarding cardiac catheterization. Like doctors across the country, they felt they were being second-guessed and micromanaged. To fight back, they developed and tested in rigorous clinical conditions a protocol for determining which patients really need catheterization. Their evidence was so compelling that the health plan had to change its policies, and family practice doctors and emergency room physicians got a new state-of-the art set of guidelines for recognizing heart attacks in the bargain (Winslow, 1997).

In the larger scheme, more physicians may be recognizing that managed care, traditionally viewed as limiting physician clinical autonomy, also holds the potential for restoring it. In seeking to develop integrated systems capable of accepting capitated payments and the risk that comes with them, many physicians are recognizing that the restoration of physician autonomy may demand the acceptance of financial accountability.

To us, the merging of autonomy with accountability is not a compromise. It is a step forward. And today, the most progressive physician groups recognize it as such. Rather than fighting insurance company oversight, they are seeking capitated payments from those insurers. The most aggressive of them— especially large medical groups and physician-hospital organizations—are seeking "full-risk" capitation, which means they accept full responsibility for all the care the patient may need. In doing so, they assume the responsibility to deliver cost-effective care. More important, as the ability to measure and compare quality improves, these integrated medical organizations should emerge as the strongest marketplace competitors. Not only will they be best positioned to deliver high quality, they will also have a greater capacity to demonstrate it.

9. TOWARD GREATER HEALTH PLAN LIABILITY: ANOTHER APPROACH TO MALPRACTICE

Health plans demand the authority to select their providers, place strong financial pressures on their physicians to practice differently than they did under fee-for-service, and make preauthorization decisions that may determine whether patients are able to obtain medical services their physicians recommend. Yet, if something goes seriously wrong with the care provided, health plans typically argue, in effect, that they had nothing to do with it—after all, only physicians practice medicine. For the most part, state and federal law, based primarily on the broad scope of the ERISA statute, has supported this health plan posture and, consequently, health plans have generally been protected against lawsuits accusing them of wrongdoing. Thus, where alleged negligence occurs, patients may have little recourse but to sue the involved physicians and other providers, even if the policies, procedures, or decisions of the plan were a major contributor to the poor outcome in a case.

In our view, managed care organizations should be liable for the policies they have and the decisions they make, provided that it can be demonstrated that these policies and decisions directly harmed a patient. For example, if a physician misses a diagnosis because the protocols imposed by the plan did not include (and the plan would not pay for) a test the physician thought should be run, the plan should be liable. If they direct patients to a surgeon with unacceptably bad outcomes on certain procedures, they should be liable for bad outcomes that result. Like physicians seeking more autonomy, plans seeking more control must accept the accountability that goes with it. Such a policy might serve as a useful deterrent against the tendency to push cost containment and limitations on access and services to a point where they might threaten a patient's well-being. And by allowing another means by which patients could seek protection, assigning managed care organizations legal liability for negligent performance might also reduce the need for some government-imposed rules on how managed care organizations deliver care.[1]

10. CONSOLIDATION VS. INTEGRATION: AN ANTITRUST CHALLENGE

Few government officials need to make as many complicated trade-off decisions as those who enforce antitrust laws. When

---

1. However, the managed care industry's concern that managed care organizations might often be viewed by juries as corporate "deep pockets" and be hit with judgements far in excess of patient injuries is a valid one. Thus, managed care organization corporate liability should be accompanied by tort reform, including reasonable limits on damage awards.

hospitals, plans, physicians, or pharmaceutical companies want to merge with or acquire one another, those officials must determine whether the consolidation will have a negative impact on competition. Even if that impact may be negative, they will still have to weigh the potential loss of competition against benefits—e.g., efficiency, lower costs, and higher quality—that the proposed consolidation may produce.

For example, a merger of two hospitals might pose a threat to competition in a region. But if the merger led to closure of some units in each, costs might be reduced. If the units closed are the ones performing at a lower standard, quality might be enhanced.

But, to date, it is clear that marketplace mergers and acquisitions have been more about achieving market power (which may threaten competition) than about the kinds of integration (making the newly merged parts work together) that might produce consumer benefit. The two hospitals alluded to here are more likely to merge for the purpose of forcing a health plan to contract with them than for the purpose of closing the poorer performer of two coronary units. Two groups of heart specialists merging into one may first think about how the merger might increase their leverage with managed care organizations and only later about how it might increase their efficiency or the quality of care they offer.

Integration, in other words, has generally lagged well behind consolidation, and its benefits may be long in coming. Before it does, the formation of hospitals into systems, of physicians into larger and larger medical groups and of plans into mega-corporations could leave many communities with but a handful of competitors and no public benefit to balance the loss of competition. The potential lesson for antitrust enforcers and courts is to place a considerable burden of proof on those seeking to demonstrate that their proposed consolidation will lead to integration and consumer benefit.

11. COMPETING ON QUALITY: THE DEVIL IN THE DETAILS

If a reputation for high quality is a marketplace loser because it attracts the highest cost cases, quality improvement will be slow in coming. Encouraging and ensuring fair competition on quality will require the implementation of two strategies.

First, there must be a means to pay plans or risk-bearing providers according to the health status or risk of the populations they service. Those that, for whatever reason, service more high-risk, high-cost individuals need to get paid more. For example, payments to plans could be adjusted according to the numbers of enrollees in the plan with specific defined diagnoses, such as diabetes or AIDS. The risk adjustment could be done prospectively, by raising or lowering payments to plans in a given year (e.g., 1997) based on diagnostic information from the previous year (in this case, 1996). Or, it could be done retrospectively, by raising or lowering payments to plans based on diagnostic information in the current year.

Until recently, most risk-adjustment strategies seemed more risky than viable. All the techniques proposed can be complex and controversial. But highly respected researchers are advocating that some risk-adjustment techniques are good enough to support large-scale demonstration projects (Newhouse, Buntin, and Chapman, 1997).

Unfortunately, the technological hurdles are not the only ones that risk-adjustment strategies must overcome. Implementing a risk-adjustment strategy entails taking some funds that would have gone to those plans or providers who enroll lower risk populations and shifting those funds to those who enroll higher risk populations. Whoever directs this redistribution—employer, insurer, coalition, or government—risk adjustment is still a zero-sum game that creates winners and losers—the worst kind of political exercise.

Second, at least until risk-adjustment mechanisms are perfected, laws that limit the ability of plans to select who they enroll and do not enroll must be vigorously enforced. Schemes that attempt to attract the healthy and/or avoid the less healthy—like trying to identify and enroll only active, healthy Medicare beneficiaries by inviting them to square dance—have to be identified, and those who implement them punished. Especially in the Medicare and Medicaid programs, where efforts to avoid enrolling high-cost individuals can get particularly aggressive, enrollment programs need to be monitored or perhaps even taken out of the hands of plans themselves.

How plans structure benefits is also worth watching. Adding a low-cost, preventive dental benefit for children may sound innocuous enough. But its purpose is probably to attract young, healthy, prevention-oriented families who may prove to be better (i.e., lower cost) risks. Offering higher deductibles may also be a strategy in the risk-selection game. The individual who accepts a $1,000 deductible is usually the healthy individual who does not anticipate high medical costs. By contrast, individuals with chronic diseases will avoid those deductibles and generally buy all the insurance they can.

Insurers will always be ahead in this game. They will always find another, new way to do what they need to do. This is the nature and problem of the insurance process.

But we need not be helpless in combating it. Giving individuals access to all plans helps. Stiff enforcement, including substantial fines and publication of those fines, can also help. So, too, can enrollment procedures—through employers or purchasing coalitions, or even government—that limit the insurer's control over the enrollment process. Some standardization of benefits, so that consumers can more easily compare plan offerings, would also be valuable. And finally, since we will never stop it all, risk-adjustment mechanisms are needed to balance the scales and neutralize the outcome. When those who enroll healthier populations are paid less per person, they may see less value in the risk-selection strategy.

12. A NATIONAL REPORT ON HEALTH CARE QUALITY

As a means of continually highlighting the search for quality improvement an agency of the federal government or independent commission should be given the responsibility of presenting a periodic, comprehensive report on quality in American health care. Such a report could focus on progress made in raising health care quality, obstacles to progress, aspects of health care quality that may require special attention, and strategies—for purchasers, providers, consumers, insurers and government—that might lead to improvements in health care quality.

The report might have the greatest potential impact if mandated in an Act of Congress. It could be assigned to any of several already existing government agencies, or to a new independent commission composed of nongovernment experts. The report might come in the form of periodic reviews on specific issues, or one annual or semiannual overview. But the overall goal ought to be the creation of a highly credible and visible analysis that had enough weight behind it to command the attention of the public and policy makers.

13. FROM TRADITIONAL REGULATION TO THE BULLY PULPIT

A few years ago, New York City consumer advocate Mark Green expressed an expansive view of consumer protection. His focus, undoubtedly somewhat controversial, was not on the resolution of individual complaints made by individual consumers, but on the creative use of press conferences and other media-oriented opportunities to reach millions of consumers with tips, warnings, and conspicuous examples of "rip-offs." This was supplemented with pats on the back for good business practices and the dissemination of information about how consumers could protect their own interests in the marketplace. To Green, consumer protection was not primarily about one-on-one grievance procedures; it was about public finger-pointing and broad-based public education. The tool of consumer protection was not a phone, or even a regulation; it was a TV camera (Green, 1991).

Effective consumer protection, we have asserted, involves more than a series of regulatory dos and don'ts. It is more than the resolution of complaints, one by one. It is, in its most aggressive and perhaps most productive form, about public education. Insurance commissioners, health officials, state consumer protection agencies, elected officials, and consumer groups must all be prepared to better inform and educate large populations of consumers about their health care choices and rights. The collection, even the resolution, of consumer complaints is of only modest value if consumers do not know which companies are getting more of them, or handling them unacceptably. Purchasing coalitions will be of no value to employers or employees if they do not know about them. New data on outcomes from high-cost, high-risk procedures in different hospitals needs to land on page one and the evening news. Just as two hospitals planning to merge may need an antitrust attorney, a good consumer-protection program will need a publicist.

The case of Mr. Christie and Take Care HMO outlined in Chapter 9 offers a good example here. Had the issue ended with the payment of hospital and surgeon's fees by Take Care, consumer education would have been virtually nonexistent. Even fining Take Care $500,000 would have had limited impact on consumers. What made the fine important was its appearance on page one of virtually every California newspaper. Real punishment could then occur in the marketplace.

Similarly, hiring consumer affairs officers to staff an 800 phone number and settle individual complaints with insurers may prove helpful, if expensive. But compiling complaint statistics and holding a press conference identifying the insurers with the highest rates of justified complaints will have far greater impact. Very likely, those insurers near the top of the list will work hard to improve their standing in next year's listing. Indeed, they are likely to be on a list of those who have made the greatest improvement in handling consumer complaints.

Such tactics must be employed judiciously, and with appropriate caveats. But, especially given the limited resources of those charged with consumer protection, emphasis must be placed on educating large numbers with small budgets. As we have already suggested, plans and providers will respond more quickly to punishment that may hurt them in the marketplace than to individualized, regulatory slaps on the wrist.

Epilogue | *Bridge Over Troubled Water*

Managed care has not yet secured the confidence of the American consumer. Far from it. Many remain concerned about the incentives and restrictions it can impose, about their loss of choice, and, most important, about the quality of care produced.

We have suggested that, in some respects at least, consumers may be wrong about managed care. If it is not as good as we think it can be, neither is it as bad as many believe it to be. We have also suggested that, in many respects, consumers may be wrong in their evaluation of and preference for the system that preceded managed care; its costs were out of control and its quality less than met the eye.

But even if consumers were to accept our analysis, they would still be far from comfortable with the new system. Achieving a real comfort level with managed care is going to require at least two developments: first, a genuine acceptance, on the part of consumers, that cost does count and that some restraints on access and choice may be necessary and, in many cases, even appropriate and beneficial; and second, demonstrable improvement in the quality of care delivered by managed care plans.

We have outlined some of the impediments to achieving these ends, and some means by which those impediments might be addressed. We have suggested that more and better government regulation may be part of the solution. But we have also argued that when it comes to demanding more quality, our main focus must be on getting more consumers more power in the marketplace. In the end, managed care plans will strive to maximize quality not because government rules force them to, but because better quality pays off in the marketplace.

If and when quality in managed care plans is demonstrably better, sizable and potentially very beneficial outcomes might result. If Americans were more comfortable with managed care—with its restrictions and its quality—they would not need to demand those kinds of arrangements (e.g., wider choice, and easier access to specialists) that drive up costs. They might get more value for their health care dollar, while still having more funds available to pursue other needs—education, higher salaries, etc.

Additionally, if managed care proved more acceptable, we would all be more comfortable with the use of managed care in the Medicaid and Medicare programs. However we choose to finance Medicare, and whatever the kinds of choices made available to Medicare beneficiaries, greater use of managed care could almost certainly reduce program costs and/or increase the benefits the program offers.

Finally, there is the lingering and socially embarrassing reality of more than 40 million Americans without insurance of any kind. Some of them can afford insurance but choose not to buy it. But for the great majority of them, not having insurance is a matter of money, and getting them insurance or some other form of adequate health care will entail help from the rest of us. If managed care can reduce the amount needed to secure care for all, society might be more willing to produce it, and the sorry reality of the uninsured would change.

And that should make us all feel better.

References

Abelson, R., "Behind the Bleeding at Oxford." *New York Times*, December 9, 1997, Dl.

"A Comparison of Consumer Choice Health Purchasing Groups." Material prepared by Institute for Health Policy Solutions, Washington, D.C., Oct., 1997.

Anders, G., *Health against Wealth: HMOs and the Breakdown of Medical Trust.* Boston: Houghton Mifflin, 1996.

Anderson, G.F., "In Search of Value: An International Comparison of Cost, Access and Outcomes." *Health Affairs*, Nov./Dec., 1997, *16*(2), 163–171.

Ayanian, J.Z., and others, "Knowledge and Practices of Generalist and Specialist Physicians Regarding Drug Therapy for Acute Myocardial Infarction." *New England Journal of Medicine*, Oct. 27, 1994, *331*(17), 1136–1142.

Azevedo, D., "Will the States Get Tough with HMOs?" *Medical Economics*, Aug. 26, 1996, 172–184.

Bates, D.W., and others, "Incidence of Adverse Drug Events in Hospitalized Patients." *Journal of the American Medical Association*, Jan. 22/29, 1997, *277*(4), 307–311.

Berenson, R.A., "Beyond Competition." *Health Affairs*, March/April 1997, *16*(2), 171–180.

Berwick, D.M., "Quality of Health Care Part 5: Payment by Capitation and the Quality of Care." *New England Journal of Medicine*, Oct. 17, 1996, *335*(16), 1227–1231.

Bradley, B., Presentation to Texas HMO Association, San Antonio, Oct. 1, 1997.

Brennan, T.A., and D.M. Berwick, *New Rules: Regulation, Markets, and the Quality of American Health Care.* San Francisco: Jossey Bass, 1996, 298–396.

Brennan, T.A., and others, "Incidence of Adverse Events and Negligence in Hospitalized Patients: Results of the Harvard Medical Practice Study I." *New England Journal of Medicine,* Feb. 7, 1991, *324*(6), 370–376.

Brink, S., and N. Shute, "Are HMOs the Right Prescription." *U.S. News and World Report,* Oct. 13, 1997, 60–67.

Burstin, H.R, S.R. Lipsitz, and T.A. Brennan, "Socio-Economic Status and Risks for Substandard Medical Care." *Journal of the American Medical Association,* Nov. 4, 1992, *268*(17), 2383–2387.

Butler, P. and K. Polzer, "Private-Sector Health Coverage: Variation in Consumer Protections under ERISA and State Law, National Health Policy Forum, Washington, D.C., June, 1966.

Center for Studying Health System Change, Issue Brief, Washington, D.C., May, 1997.

Chassin M.R., "Quality of Health Care Part 3: Improving the Quality of Care." *New England Journal of Medicine,* October 1996, 225(14) 1060–1062.

———, "Assessing Strategies for Quality Improvement," *Health Affairs,* May/June 1997.

Chassin, M.R., and others, "Does Inappropriate Use Explain Geographic Variations in the Use of Health Services? A Study of Three Procedures." *Journal of the American Medical Association,* 1987, *258*(18), 2533–2537.

Church, G.J., "Twin Cities' Friendly Plans." *Time,* Apr. 14, 1997, 36–39.

Claxton, G., and others, "Public Policy Issues in Nonprofit Conversions: An Overview." *Health Affairs,* Mar./Apr., 1997, *16*(3), 9–28.

Crozier, D.A., "National Medical Care Spending." *Health Affairs,* Fall 1984, *3*(3), 108–120.

Dallek, G., "HMO Consumers at Risk," *Families,* USA. Washington, D.C., July 1966.

Darling, H. "Book Review: Are HMOs Really Dangerous to Your Health?" *Health Affairs,* July/Aug. 1997, *16*(4), 277–279.

Davis, K. and C. Schoen, "Managed Care, Choice, and Patient Satisfaction," The Commonwealth Fund, New York, August, 1997.

Dial, T.H., and others, *HMO and PPO Industry Profile, 1995–96.* Washington, D.C.: American Association of Health Plans, 1996.

Eisenberg, D.M., and others, "Unconventional Medicine in the United States: Prevalence, Costs, and Patterns of Use." *New England Journal of Medicine,* Jan. 28, 1993, *328*(4), 246–252.

Enthoven A.C., "Consumer Choice Health Plan: A National Health Insurance Proposal Based on Regulated Competition in the Private Sector," *The New England Journal of Medicine* (23 and 30 March 1978): 650–658 and 709–720.

Enthoven, A.C. and S.J. Singer, "Markets and Collective Action in Regulating Managed Care," *Health Affairs,* November/December 1997, 16(b) 26–32.

Epstein, A.M., "The Role of Quality Measurement in a Competitive Marketplace." Presentation at Harvard Conference on Strategic Alliances, Boston, Nov. 18, 1997.

Etheredge, L., and S. Jones, *Consumers, Gag Rules, and Health Plans: Strategies for a Patient-Focused Market.* Washington, D.C.: George Washington University, 1997.

Fox, P.D., "An Overview of Managed Care." In P.R. Kongstvedt, *The Managed Health Care Handbook,* third edition. Gaithersburg, MD: Aspen Publishers, 1996, 3–5.

Fuchs, V.R., *Who Shall Live? Health, Economics, and Social Choice."* New York: Basic Books, 1974.

Gabel, J.R., "Ten Ways HMOs Have Changed During the 1990s." *Health Affairs,* May/June, 1997 *16*(3) 134–145.

———, Interview with author. Washington, D.C., July, 1997.

Gabel, J.R., and K.A. Hunt, *Health Benefits in 1996, Executive Summary.* Washington, D.C.: KPMG, 1996.

Gabel, J.R., P.B. Ginsburg, and K.A. Hunt, "Small Employers and Their Health Benefits, 1988–1996: An Awkward Adolescence. *Health Affairs,* September/October, 1997, 16(5).

Gazmararian J.A., and others, "Maternity Experiences In A Managed Care Organization."*Health Affairs,* May/June 1997.

Gold, M.R., and others, "A National Survey of the Arrangements Managed-Care Plans Make with Physicians." *New England Journal of Medicine,* Dec. 21, 1995, *333*(25), 1678–1683.

Governance Committee, The, *The Grand Alliance,* The Advisory Board, Washington, D.C., 1993.

Gray, B.H., and M.J. Field (Eds.), *Controlling Costs and Changing Patient Care? The Role of Utilization Management.* Washington, D.C.: Institute of Medicine, 1989.

Green, Mark, Interview with author, January 1991.

Greenspan, A.M., and others, "Incidence of Unwarranted Implantation of Permanent Cardiac Pacemakers in a Large

Medical Population." *New England Journal of Medicine*, Jan. 21, 1988, *318*(3), 158–163.

Guadagnoli, R., and others, "Variation in the Use of Cardiac Procedures After Acute Myocardial Infarction." *New England Journal of Medicine,* Aug. 31, 1995, *333*(9), 573–578.

Guglielmo, W.J., "Is the Classic Staff-Model HMO a Dinosaur?" *Medical Economics*, Nov. 25, 1996, 46–50.

Health Care Advisory Board. Emerging from Shadow. Washington, D.C.: Advisory Board Company, 1995.

————, *The Resurgence of Choice*, The Advisory Board Company, Washington, D.C., 1996.

"Healthcare CEO Compensation Jumped 25%." *Jenks Healthcare Business Report*. Business Wire, Sept. 26, 1997.

Health Care Financing Review. "Table 116: Gross Domestic Product, National Health Expenditures, and Federal and State and Local Government Expenditures and Average Annual Percent Change: United States, Selected Years, 1960–95." *Health Care Financing Review* 18(1), 246. Washington, D.C.: Health Care Financing Administration, Fall 1996.

Herbert, B., "A Chance to Survive." *New York Times,* July 4, 1997, A19.

Herzlinger, R., *Market Driven Health Care: Who Wins, Who Loses in the Transformation of America's Largest Industry*. Boston: Addison-Wesley, 1997.

Hilzenrath, D.S., "HMO's Prescription for Change: Flexibility." *Washington Post*, Oct. 20, 1997, 1, 12.

————, "What's Left to Squeeze," *Washington Post*, July 6, 1997.

Iglehart, J.K., "Interview: State Regulation of Managed Care: NAIC President Josephine Musser." *Health Affairs*, Nov./Dec., 1997, *15*(6), 36–45.

Jensen, G.A., and others, "The New Dominance of Managed Care: Insurance Trends in the 1990s." *Health Affairs*, Jan./Feb., 1997, *16*(5), 125–136.

Jollis, J.G., and others, "Outcome of Acute Myocardial Infarction According to the Specialty of the Admitting Physician." *New England Journal of Medicine*, Dec. 19, 1996, *335*(25), 1880–1887.

Katz, J., *The Silent World of Doctor and Patient*. New York: New York Free Press, 1984.

Kerr, C., Untitled presentation, Conference on Health Care Purchasing, the Alpha Center, Washington, D.C. July 11, 1997.

Kilborn, P.T., "Trend to Managed Care is Unpopular, Surveys Find," *New York Times*, Sept. 28, 1997.

————, "Workers Getting Greater Freedom in Health Plans." *New York Times*, Aug. 17, 1997.

Kleinman, L.C., and others, "The Medical Appropriateness of Tympanostomy Tubes Proposed for Children Younger than 16 Years in the United States." *Journal of the American Medical Association*, Apr. 27, 1994, *271*(16), 1250–1255.

Kosecoff, J., and others, "Effects of a National Institutes of Health Consensus Development Program on Physician Practice." *Journal of the American Medical Association*, Nov. 20, 1987, *258*(19), 2708–2713.

KPMG, "Health Benefits in 1996," KPMG Peat Marwick, Washington D.C., October, 1996.

Lewis, N.A., "Agency Facing Revolt After Report: Enraged Back Surgeons Recruiting Republicans for a Battle." *New York Times*, Sept. 14, 1995.

Lipson, D.J., and L.M. De Sa, "Purchasers." *Health Affairs*, Summer 1996, *15*(2), 62–76.

Localio, A.R., and others, "Relation between Malpractice Claims and Adverse Events Due to Negligence." *New England Journal of Medicine*, Jul. 25, 1991, *325*(10), 245–251.

Lomas, J., and others, "Do Practice Guidelines Guide Practice: The Effect of a Consensus Statement on the Practice of Physicians." *New England Journal of Medicine*, Nov. 9, 1989, *321*(19), 1306–1311.

Lubalin, J.S., and L. Harris-Kojetin, "What Do Consumers Want and Need to Know in Making Health Care Choices?" Presented at Conference on Health Care Choices Facing Consumers, sponsored by Robert Wood Johnson Foundation, Washington, D.C., Nov. 19, 1997.

Luft, H.S., "Addressing the Quality of Care in an Increasingly Competitive Environment," Presentation to the National Roundtable on Health Care Quality, Institute of Medicine, Spring 1997.

McLaughlin, C.G., "Health Care Consumers: Choices and Constraints." Presented at Conference on Health Care Choices Facing Consumers, sponsored by Robert Wood Johnson Foundation, Washington, D.C., Nov. 19, 1997.

"Medicaid Facts," The Kaiser Commission on the Future of Medicaid, Washington, D.C., 1996.

"The Medicare Program, Managed Care," The Kaiser Family Foundation, Washington, D.C., April 1997.

Merrill, J.C., "Growth in National Expenditures: Additional Analyses." *Health Affairs*, Winter, 1985, *4*(4), 91–97.

Millenson, M.L., *Beyond the Managed Care Backlash*. Washington, D.C.: Progressive Policy Institute, June, 1997a.

———, *Demanding Medical Excellence: Doctors and Accountability in the Information Age*. Chicago: University of Chicago Press, 1997b.

Miller, R.H. and H.S. Luft, "Does Managed Care Lead to Better or Worse Quality of Care?" *Health Affairs*, Sept./Oct. 1997, *16*(5), 7–25.

———, "Managed Care Plan Performance Since 1980." *Journal of the American Medical Association*, 1994, *271*(19), 1512–1519.

Moskowitz, D.B., *Perspectives on the Marketplace*. Washington, D.C.: Faulkner and Gray, 1997.

National Committee for Quality Assurance, Press release, Washington, D.C., October 1, 1997.

Neustadt, R.E., *Presidential Power*. New York: Wiley, 1960.

Newcomer, L.N., "Measures of Trust in Health Care." *Health Affairs*, Jan./Feb. 1997, *16*(1), 50–51.

Newhouse, J.P., M. Beeuwkes Buntin, and J.D. Chapman, "Risk Adjustment and Medicare: Taking a Closer Look." *Health Affairs*, Sept./Oct., 1997, *16*(5), 26–43.

Pacific Currents, San Francisco: Pacific Business Group on Health, 1997.

Pear, R., "The Tricky Business of Keeping Doctors Quiet, *New York Times*, September 22, 1996.

Pearlstein, S., "Turning to a Specialist to Curb Rising Health Care Costs." *Washington Post*, Oct. 23, 1997, C1,7.

Pilote, L., and others, "Regional Variation Across the United States in the Management of Acute Myocardial Infarction." *New England Journal of Medicine*, Aug. 31, 1995, *333*(9), 565–572.

Polzer, K., and P.A. Butler, "Employee Health Plan Protections Under ERISA." *Health Affairs*, Sept./Oct., 1997, *16*(5), 93–102.

Physician Payment Review Commission, Annual Report to Congress, Appendix D. Physician Payment Review Commission, 1995.

"Public Perceptions and Experiences with Managed Care." Poll commissioned by the Managed Health Care Improvement Task Force, California, 1997.

Raible, R., Interview with Walter Zelman, Washington, D.C. September, 1997.

Reinhardt, Uwe, Speech to National Health Care Management, Washington, D.C., May 1, 1997.

Remler D.K., Donelan K., R.J. Blendon, G.D. Lundberg, L.L. Leape, D.R. Calkins, K. Binns, and J.P. Newhouse, "What Do Managed Care Plans Do To Affect Care: Results from a Survey of Physicians" *Inquiry* 34: 196–204 Fall 1997.

Rich M.W., and others, "A Multidisciplinary Intervention to Prevent the Readmission of Elderly Patients with Congestive Heart Failure." *New England Journal of Medicine*, Nov. 2, 1995, 333(18), 1190–1195.

Robinson, J.C., and L.P. Casalino, "Vertical Integration and Organizational Networks in Health Care." *Health Affairs*, Spring, 1996, *15*(1), 7–22.

Rodwin, M.A., "Consumer Protection and Managed Care: Issues, Reform Proposals, and Trade-Offs," *Houston Law Review*, Vol 32, Number 5, 1996.

Salkever D. and T.W. Bice, "Hospital Certificate of Need Controls: Impact on Investment, Costs and Use," Washington DC: American Enterprise Institute, 1979.

Schuster M.A., E.A. McGlynn, and R.H. Brook, "Why the Quality of U.S. Health Care Must Be Improved." Manuscript prepared for The National Coalition on Health Care. Rand, Santa Monica, Cal., Oct. 1997.

Siren, P.B. and G.L. Laffel, "Quality Management in Managed Care." In P.R. Kongstveldt. *The Managed Health Care Handbook*, third edition. Gaithersburg, MD: Aspen, 1996.

Sloan F.A., "Containing Health Expenditures Lessons Learned from Certificate-of-Need Programs," in *Cost, Quality, and Access in Health Care*, Sloan F.A., Blumstein J.F., Perrin J.M., Editors, Jossey-Bass, San Francisco, 1988.

Soumerai, S.B., and others, "Adverse Outcomes of Underuse of b-Blockers in Elderly Survivors of Acute Myocardial Infarction." *Journal of the American Medical Association*, Jan. 8, 1997, *277*(2), 115–121.

Starr, P., *The Social Transformation of American Medicine*. New York: Basic Books, 1982.

"The State of Quality in Managed Care." National Committee for Quality Assurance, Washington, D.C., 1997.

Sullivan, C.B., and T. Rice, "The Health Insurance Picture in 1990." *Health Affairs,* Summer 1991, *10*(2), 104–115.

Ullman, and others, *Health Affairs*, May/June 1997, *16*(3), 209–217.

Ware, J.E., and others, "Differences in 4-Year Health Outcomes for Elderly and Poor, Chronically Ill Patients Treated in HMO and Fee-for-Service Systems." *Journal of the American Medical Association,* Oct. 2, 1996, *276*(13), 1039–1047.

Wells, K.B., and others, "Detection of Depressive Disorder for Patients Receiving Prepaid or Fee-for-Service Care: Results from the Medical Outcomes Study." *Journal of the American Medical Association*, Dec. 15, 1989, *262*(23), 3298–3302.

Wennberg, J., "Dealing with Medical Practice Variations: A Proposal for Action." *Health Affairs*, Summer 1984, *3*(2), 6–32.

Winslow, R., "Heal Thyself." *Wall Street Journal*, October 23, 1997, R15.

Zall, R.J., R. Belfort, and S. Berkow, *Who Should Protect Managed Care Consumers*? New York: Zall and Bernstein LLP, June 1997.

Zelman, W.A., *The Changing Health Care Marketplace*: *Private Ventures, Public Interests*. San Francisco: Josey Bass, 1996.

Index

Abelson, R., 144
access to services, 167–68
access to specialists, 111–12, 123, **124**
accountability, 195–96
   physicians, 38–39
accreditation, 154–55
acquisitions, 13, 113, 140–41, 196–97
administrative vs. medical costs, 169–70
advice lines, 91
Aetna, 111, 113, 182
Agency for Health Care Policy and Research (AHCPR), 88–89
AIDS, 175
alternative therapies, 45
AMA (American Medical Association), 29, 32, 37, 50–51
American Hospital Association, 32
American Medical Association (AMA), 29, 32, 37, 50–51
Anders, George, 107
Anderson, G.F., 1
anecdotes, 102–3, 105–8
Anthem, 113
anticriticism clauses, 126
anti-managed care legislation, 104–5, 120–21, 129
antitrust laws, 51, 196–97

any willing provider, 117, 174, 180
appeals process, 84, 164–65
arbitration, 177
asthma management program, 10, 42, 94–97, 98
atrial flutter, 7–8
at-risk patients, 96
at-risk physicians, 110, 124, 128, 169
attacks on managed care, 10–12
authority vs. persuasion, 160–62
Ayanian, J.Z., 42, 77
Azevedo, D., 163–64

backlash, 10–12, 102–18
   choice, access, and quality, 111–12
   consumer concerns, 108–11
   greed factor, 112–15
   horror stories, 105–8
   physicians, 115–17
back-pain guidelines, 89
Balanced Budget Act, 62, 170
bashing. *See* backlash
Bates, D.W., 44
benchmark HMOs, 153, **154**
beneficiary costs, 156–57
benefit carve-outs, 97–98
Berenson, Robert A., 7, 115, 142

Note: **Boldface** locators indicate a chart; locators followed by *n* indicate footnotes.

Berwick, D.M., 10, 79, 167
beta blockers, 42, 132
Bice, T.W., 31
Bioethics, Center for, University of Minnesota, 130
blaming managed care, 121–23
Blue Cross, 111, 182
Blue Cross and Blue Shield, 51
Bradley, B., 153
breast cancer screening, 191
Brennan, T.A., 39, 43, 167
Brink, S., 123
Brook, Robert, H., 134
Buntin, M. Beeuwkes, 198
Burstin, H.R., 39
business comparisons, 109, **109**
Butler, P., 175–76

CABGs (coronary artery bypass grafts), 70
California, 163–64
    delivery systems, 150–51
    Health Insurance Purchasing Cooperative (HIPC), 183
    health plans, **190–91**
    model plan, 183
    performance reports, 189, **190–91**
call-in lines, 91
capitation, 79–82, 83
    arrangements, 169
    benefits of, 128–29
    full-risk, 195
    payment strategies, 124–25
cardiac catheterization, 82–85, 194
cardiologists, 82–85, 194–95
Carter, Jimmy, 31–32, 33
carve-outs, 97–98
case managers, 76–78
case study, catheterization, 82–85
catastrophically ill, 93–94
catheterization, 82–85, 194
Center for Bioethics, University of Minnesota, 130

Center for Studying Health System Change, 113, 147–48
CEO compensation, 113–14
certificates of need, 30
cervical cancer screening, 190
Chapman, J.D., 198
Chassin, M.R., 6, 41, 42
childhood immunization, 190
choice, integration, quality, 188–89
Choice Care, 126
choice of delivery system, 182–83
choice of plan, 145–49
choice of physician, 111–12, 141–45
choice vs. cost, **69**
Christie, Harry, 177, 201
chronically ill, 93–94, 130, 131–32, **131**, 134
Cigna, 111
clinical practice guidelines, 83, 85, 88–90, 96
Clinton, Bill, 105
Clinton plan, 4, 19, 32, 62–63
coalition strategies, 183–86
collaborative relationships, 85, 87, 97, 99
Columbia/HCA, 112–13
competition, 14–15, 139–40
competition on quality, 197–99
competition vs. regulation, 63
congestive heart failure, 94, 97
Congress, 26, 32, 104–5
consolidation vs. integration, 196–97
consumer considerations
    backlash, 102–18
    choice, 179–82
    complaints, 200–201
    concerns, 108–11
    cost-consciousness, 186–88, **187**
    fears, 11–12
    groups, 185–86
    as losers, 18
    public education, 200–201
    satisfaction, 134–35

consumer protection, 160–62, 162–64, 200–201
  and self-insured employers, 175–76
consumer protection enforcement, 163–64
  access and quality, 166–68
  delivery systems, 170–72
  disclosure, 165–66
  due process, 164–65
  Employee Retirement Income Security Act (ERISA), 174–77
  financial arrangements, 168–70
  Medicaid and Medicare, 172–73
  provider protections, 173–74
  regulatory and market-based powers, 177–78
consumer protection legislation, 120–21
"Consumer Reports," 123, 181
contracting, selective, 69–72, 83
contribution strategies, employer, 186–87, **187**
conventional health insurance, 45, **58**, 59, 61. *See also* fee-for-service; traditional insurance
coordination of care, 99–101
coronary angiography, 41–42
coronary artery bypass grafts (CABGs), 70
corporatization of medicine, 112–15
corticosteroids, 96
cost-conscious consumers, 186–88, **187**
cost controls, 99
  in Nixon Administration, 30–31
  in other countries, 1, 27
  selective contracting, 69–72
  and tools of managed care, 86
cost cutting, 53–55
cost inflation, 1, 16, 20, 30, 32
cost-quality trade-offs, 107–8
costs, 1–4, 2, 16
  and government, 18, 25–26
  soaring, 28–30, 61

cost savings, 120–21
cost trade-offs, 120–21, 186–87, **187**
cost unconsciousness, 18–19, 21
cost vs. choice, **69**
cottage industry, 37–39, 42, 46
  payment system, 78–79
  See also fee-for-service; traditional insurance; traditional medicine
Crowley, Dan, 113
Crozier, D.A., 33
customer choice, 179–82
customers, best, 109, **109**
customer satisfaction, 134–35

Dallek, G., 163, 166
Dana Farber Cancer Institute, 44
Davis, K., 157
D.C. IPA (District of Columbia, Independent Physicians Association), 156
DEC (Digital Equipment Corporation), 189
decision-making, shared, 92
delivery systems, 149–51
  choices of, 182–83
  local, 171
  new, 170–72
Demanding Medical Excellence, (Millenson), 95
demand management strategy, 91–93
De Sa, L.M., 155
diabetes, 94, 97
diabetic retinal exams, 190
Dial, T.H., 59
Digital Equipment Corporation (DEC), 189
disclosure, 165–66
disease management, 94–97
District of Columbia, Independent Practice Associations (D.C. IPA), 156

doctors. *See* physicians
Doctor's Dilemma, The, (Shaw), 6
dosing errors, 44
due process, 164–65

educating consumers, 200–201
Eisenberg, D.M., 45
elderly, the, 131–32, **131**, 172–73
electronic information age, 189–93
electronic medical records, 42
Ellwood, Paul, 52
emergency room (ER), 167
emergency room visits, 96
Emphesys, 113
employee considerations
    cost-consciousness, 186–88, **187**
    plan choices, 145–49, **146**,
        179–82
    polls, 140
    surveys, 146
Employee Retirement Income Secu-
    rity Act, (ERISA), 174–77, 196
employer considerations
    contribution methods, 186–87,
        187
    health care origins, 20–21
    HMOs, 53–54
    premiums, 17, 57
    as purchaser, 180
    self-insured, 18n, 23, 57–59,
        175–76
    surveys, 140
    and value, 139–40
enforcement, consumer protec-
    tion, 163–64
enrollees
    high-cost, 109–10, 174
    high-risk, 156–57, 198–99
enrollee selection, 198–99
enrollment, 11, 55, **56**, 57, 59
    choices, 188–89
    processes, 198–99
Enthoven, A.C., 26, 120
ER (emergency room), 167

ERISA (Employee Retirement
    Income Security Act), 174–77, 196
errors, medical, 43–45
Etheredge, L., 126, 157
ethics, 36–37, 46, 194
evidence-based standards, 41
evolution of managed care, 49–63
    Clinton plan, 62–63
    diversification, 55–57
    health maintenance organiza-
        tions, 51–55
    from minority to majority,
        60–61
    new products, 57–59
    opposition, 50–51
    trends, 61–62
executive pay, 113–14
expenditures, 16

Fallon Clinic, 152, 168
fears, 123–26, 133–34
Federal Employee Health Benefits
    (FEHB), 185, 186
federal government
    cost controls, 31–32
    cost increases, 26–27, 28–30
    role, 176–77
federal legislation, 105. *See also*
    anti-managed care legislation
fee-for-service, 9–10, 84
    care comparisons, 129–32
    costs, 120
    and disease management, 95
    failures, 16–34
    flaws, 1–8
    and HMOs, 52
    medications, 77
    payment system, 78–79
    quality, 35–48
    See also cottage industry; tradi-
        tional insurance
FEHB (Federal Employee Health
    Benefits), 185, 186
Field, M.J., 74
financial arrangements, 168–70

financial incentives, 79–82, 83
  and clinical decision making,
    127
  in Medicare, 33
for-profit plans, 112–15, **114**
Fortune 500 companies, 175
Foundation Health Plan, 113
Fox, P.D., 49
fragmentation, 6–8
Fuchs, Victor R., 23
full-risk capitation, 195. *See also*
  capitation

Gabel, J.R., 54, 120, 154
gag clauses/laws, 125–26, 166
gatekeeper physicians, 84–85
gatekeepers, 9, 76–78, 84
Gazmararian, J.A., 168
Geisinger, 152
General Motors (GM), 153–54, **154**
general practitioners, 76–77. *See*
  also physicians
Ginsburg, P.B., 120
GM (General Motors), 153–54, **154**
Governance Committee, 80
government and costs, 18, 25–26
government involvement, 192,
  193, 199–200
government spending, 26–27
Gray, B.H., 74
greed factor, 112–15
Green, Mark, 200
Greenspan, A.M., 6
grievance procedures, 163, 177–78
Group Health Association, 50–51
Group Health Cooperative, 49
Group Health of Puget Sound, 149
group HMOs, 67–68, **67**. *See also*
  HMOS; MCOs
group practice, prepaid, 49–51, 52
Guadagnoli, R., 42, 82
gynecologic services, 78

Harris and Associates Polls, 103
Harvard Community Health Plan.
  See Harvard Pilgrim Health Plan

Harvard Medical Practice Study, 43
Harvard Medical School, 41
Harvard Pilgrim Health Plan
  (formerly Harvard Community
  Health Plan), 95–96, 98–99
Health against Wealth: HMOs and the
  Breakdown of Medical Trust
  (Anders), 107
Health Care Advisory Board, 73,
  142–43
health care costs. *See* costs
"Health Care Financing Review," 30
health care organizations. *See*
  HMOs; MCOs
health care reports, 129–34, 189–
  92, **190–91**, 199–200
health care spending, 1–4, **2**
health care trade-offs, 188–89
health care vs. medical care, 45–46
Health Institute of the New
  England Medical Center, 131
health insurance. *See* conventional
  health insurance; traditional
  insurance
Health Insurance Plan (HIP) of New
  York, 49–50, 51, 55, 107
health maintenance organizations
  (HMOs). *See* HMOs
Healthplan Employer Data and
  Information Set (HEDIS), 90–91
health planning, 30–31
HealthSource Corporation, 113
Health System Change, Center for
  Studying, 113, 147–48
heart attacks, 41, 82–85, 132, 195
HEDIS (Healthplan Employer Data
  and Information Set), 90–91
Henry Ford System, 149
Herbert, Bob, 105
Herzlinger, R., 98
high-cost patients, 109–10, 174
high-risk enrollees, 156–57, 198–99
Hilzenrath, D.S., 103, 113
HIP (Health Insurance Plan) of New
  York, 49–50, 51, 55, 107

HIPC (California Health Insurance Purchasing Cooperative), 49–51, 183–84
HIV, 22
HMO Act of 1973, 52, 55
HMO backlash, 102–18
"HMO Consumers at Risk," 105
HMOs (health maintenance organizations)
  banned, 51
  benchmark, 153, **154**
  care comparison, 129–32
  fines, 177
  horror stories, 102–3, 105–8
  organization of, 67–68, **67**
  plan rankings, 147
  premises of, 66
  rise of, 49–63
  teamwork, 87, 99
  traditional group staff model, 152
  types of, 65–66
  See also MCOs
HMO staff model, teamwork, 87
HMO statutes, 163–64
horror stories, 102–3, 105–8
hospital admissions, 96
Hospital Cost Containment legislation, 32, 33
hospital days, 73
hospitalization rates, 54, **54**
hospitals, general vs. specialized, **71**
hospital utilization rates, 73
hotlines, 91
Humana, 111, 113
Hunt, K.A., 120
hysterectomies, 40

Iglehart, J.K., 177
improvement recommendations, 179–201
incentive payments, 79–82
independent practice associations (IPAs), 56–57, 60, 67–68, **67**
individual complaints, 200–201

information, medical, 42–43
information availability, plan, 189–93
informed consent, 46
insurance premiums, 3. *See also* premiums
insurance process, 199
insurance regulations, 58
insurance system, old, 1–8, 16–34
insurers' denial rates, 123
insurer tasks, **172**
integrated delivery systems, 170–71
Integrated Healthcare Report, 143
integration of care, 10, 78–79, 99–101
  and capitation, 81–82
  and quality, 152, 188–89
  vs. consolidation, 196–97
Intermountain Health Care, 152
Internal Revenue Service (IRS), 20
invisible hand, 19
IPAs (independent practice associations), 56–57, 60, 67–68, **67**
IRS (Internal Revenue Service), 20

Jensen, G.A., 112
Johnson, Lyndon, 16, 26, 29
Johnson Administration, 29
Jollis, J.G., 77
Jones, S., 126

Kaiser. *See* Kaiser Permanente
Kaiser Family Foundation, 103, 113
Kaiser Permanente, 49, 51, 55, 111, 143, 182
Katz, J., 46
Kerr, C., 75, 182
Kilborn, P.T., 103
Kleinman, L.C., 6
Kosecoff, J., 90

Laffel, G.L., 88
large case management, 93–94

large medical groups, 195
Lawrence, David, 143
Leape, Lucian, 43
legislation. *See* anti-managed care
  legislation; federal legislation;
  hospital cost containment
  legislation
Lehman, Betsy, 44
Leitman, Robert, 103
length-of-stay laws, 168
leverage, 53
Lewis, N.A., 89
liability, 195–96
  hospital, 38–39
  and utilization management,
  74–75
Lipsitz, S.R., 39
Lipson, D.J., 155
local delivery systems, 171
Localio, A.R., 39
logic of managed care, 8–10, 65–66,
  134, 137
logic vs. reality, 98–101
Lomas, J., 90
loss-ratio numbers, 169–70
Lovelace, 152
low back pain, 89
Luft, H.S., 129–30, 130n, 134, 156

Maine statutes, 163
malpractice, 38–39
managed care organizations. *See*
  MCOs
managed competition, 26
managing patients, 91–93
market controls, 25–26
market forces, 23–25
marketing strategies, 165
marketplace competition, 14, 20,
  63, 126–128, 138, 139
Maryland, rate-setting in, 31
Mayo Clinic, 111, 149, 152, 155
MCOs (managed care organizations)
  accountability, 195–96

backlash, 102–18
consumer concerns, 108–11
coordination and integration, 99
enrollment, 53, 55, 55n, **56**
history of, 49–51
liability, 195–96
loss of physician domination,
  53–55
and Nixon Administration,
  51–52
organizational capacity, 91–93
plan rankings, 147
product choices, 60
teamwork, 87, 99
track record, 119–36
types of, 66
See also HMOs
measuring quality, 153–55
media coverage, 102–3, 105–8,
  200–201
Medicaid, 26, 55
costs, 25
definition, 10
enrollment in HMOs, 55, 61–62,
  62
high-risk enrollees, 198–99
and managed care, 172–73
and state controls, 29
"Medicaid Facts," 61
medical associations, 173
medical care vs. health care, 45–46
"Medical Economics," 164
medical education, 45
medical integrity, 36–37, 46–48
medical loss ratios, 115
medically necessary, 73–75
medical mistakes/errors, 12, 43–45
medical records, electronic, 42
medical science, 22–23
Medicare, 32–34, 172–73
beneficiaries, 61, 131
cost review, 156
costs, 25
enrollment in HMOs, 55, 61–62,
  62
fixed fees, 33

Medicare (*continued*)
  high-risk enrollees, 198–99
  origins of, 26, 28–30
  payment system, 18
  quality of care, 131
  unnecessary procedures, 8
Medicare model, new, 182–83
Medicare 1997 reforms, 173
Medicare patients and heart
  attacks, 41–42
"Medicare Program, The," 61
medication errors, 44
medicine, region by region, 40–41
mental health services, 97–98, 129
mergers, 13, 113, 140–41, 196–97
Merrill, J.C., 16, 32
MetraHealth, 113
Miles, Steven, 130
Millenson, Michael L., 37, 53, 92,
  96
    Demanding Medical Excellence, 95
Miller, R.H., 129–30, 130n, 134
minimum-loss ratios, 169
Minnesota model, 163, 183
mistakes, 12, 43–45
Moskowitz, D.B., 189
multidisciplinary approaches,
  96–97

National Committee of Quality
  Assurance (NCQA), 132, 189
  report card, 90–91
  "State of Managed Care Quality,
    The," 132–33
National Health Policy Forum, 175
National Institutes of Health, 96
national report, 199–200
NCQA (National Committee of
  Quality Assurance), 90–91, 132,
  189
  "State of Managed Care Quality,
    The," 132–33
negligence, 43–45
network concerns, 143–45

network HMOs, 67–68, **67**. *See also*
  HMOs
network physicians, 69–72, **142.**
  See also physicians
networks, physician and hospital,
  142–45, **142**
Neustadt, R.E., 162
Newcomer, L.N., 47
New England Medical Center,
  Health Institute of the, 131
Newhouse, J.P., 198
New Jersey statutes, 163
New Jersey Blue Cross, 113
newsletters, 92
New York Hospital, 107
New York State, program monitor-
  ing, 192
New York statutes, 163
Nixon, Richard, 16, 25, 33
  and price controls, 30–31
Nixon Administration, 51–52
nonprofit plans, 112–13
Northern California's Health Plan
  of the Redwoods, 111
North Shore Hospital (New York),
  107
nurse advice lines, 91

O'Kane, Margaret, 132
old insurance system, 6–8, 16–34.
  See also conventional health
  insurance; traditional insurance
oncology, 98
open heart surgery, 192
opposition to managed care, 5, 50–
  51
organized medicine, 50–51
oversight, physician, 38–39. *See also*
  physicians
overutilization, 84
Oxford Health Plan, 143, 144–45

"Pacific Currents," 184
paid per procedure, 84. *See also* fee-
  for-service

paternalism, 36, 46
patient-first ethic, 116–17, 194
patients
    catastrophically and chronically ill, 93–94
    participation, 91–93
    trust, 38, 47
payment strategies, 9–10
Pear, R., 126
Pearlstein, S., 70
peer review, 39
peptic ulcers, 42
performance reports, 129–34, 189–92, **190–91**, 199–200. *See also* track record
per member per month (PMPM), 79–80, 82
persuasion vs. authority, 160–62
physician-hospital organizations, 195
physician-patient communications, 125–26
Physician Payment Review Commission, 175
physicians
    accountability, 38–39
    appeals, 84
    autonomy, 44, 46, 100–101, 115–17, 195
    backlash, 115–17
    choice, 111–12, 141–45
    criticisms, 104
    domination, 53–55
    financial risk, 124
    in HMOs, 68
    leadership, 193–95
    oversupply, 26–27
    in PPOs, 67–68
    and utilization management, 74–75
physicians at-risk, 110, 169
physician selection, 69–72
physicians in networks, 69–72, **142**
plan choice, 145–49
plan liability, 195–96
plans, growth of, **58**

PMPM (per member per month), 79–80, 82
point of service (POS) option, 57, **58**, 59, 60
Polzer, K., 175–76
poor, the, 132, 134, 172–73
POS (point of service) option, 57, **58**, 59, 60
potential of managed care, 12–15
PPOs (preferred provider organizations), 57–59, **58**
    organization of, 67–68, **67**
practice guidelines/statements, 83, 85, 88–90, 96
practice variations, 39–42, **40**
practice vs. theory, 12–14
preauthorizations, 53, 73–75, 76. *See also* gatekeepers
preferred provider organizations (PPOs), 57–59, **58**
    organization of, 67–68, **67**
pre-managed care, 1–4, 6–8
premiums, 120–21, **144**
    higher, 22
    paid up front, 18–19
    pre-managed care, 1–4, **3**
    and rise of managed care, 50, 54–55, 57
prenatal care, 191
prepaid group practice, 49–51, 52
prepaid health plans, 49–51, 52
prepayment, 9, 78–82
press coverage, 102–3, 105–8, 200–201
preventable errors, 43–45
preventive care, 45–46, 78–79
price competition, 53–55, 63, 139–40
price controls, 30–31
primary care physicians, 9, **81**, 124, **124**, 189. *See also* physicians
procedures, invasive, 6
procedures, unnecessary, 6–8, 73
proconsumer legislation, 104–5. *See also* anti-managed care legislation

professionalism, 36–37, 41, 46–48
profits, 113–15
proponents of managed care, 5
Prospective Payment System, 33
prostate cancer, 92
prostatectomies, 40
provider, any willing, 117, 174, 180
provider initiative, 32
provider protections, 173–74
providers, 4, 27–28
provider-sponsored organizations
    (PSOs), 170–71, **172**, 182
Prudential, 182
PSOs (provider-sponsored organiza-
    tions), 170–71, **172**, 182
"Public Perceptions," 104
public education, 200–201
public relations, 121–23, **122.** *See
    also* press coverage
purchaser power strategies, 183–86
purchasers, weak, 21–22
purchasing coalitions, 183–86, 192
pyrrhic victory, 31–32

quality, demonstrating, 153–55
quality and access, 166–68
quality and integration, 152,
    188–89
quality and mergers, 140–41
quality assessments, 153–55
quality assurance, 88, 90–91,
    166–67
    medical or administrative cost,
    169
"Quality Compass," 189
quality competition, 197–99
quality-cost trade-offs, 107–8
quality improvement, 87–101,
    151–52
quality improvement programs,
    88–91
quality improvement recommenda-
    tions, 179–201
    choice of delivery systems, 182
    competition strategies, 197–99

    consolidation vs. integration,
    196–97
    cost-conscious consumers,
    186–88, **187**
    employee choice, 179–82
    health care trade-offs, 188–89
    information revolution, 189–93
    physician leadership, 193–95
    plan liability, 195–96
    public education, 200–201
    purchaser power strategies,
    183–86
    reporting, 199–200
quality in traditional medicine,
    35–48
quality of care, 129–34, 134
quality reporting, 199–200
quality selling, 155–58
quality strategies, 197–99
quality vs. choice, 145

Raible, Robert, 102–3
raising quality, 151–52
Reagan, Ronald, 32
Reagan Administration, 33
reality vs. logic, 98–101
recommendations, 179–201
referrals, 37, 123, **124**
regulation vs. competition, 63
regulatory framework, 162–64
regulatory vs. market-based power,
    177–78
Reinhardt, Uwe, 139
Remler, D.K., 123
reporting, 199–200. *See also* perfor-
    mance reports
Rice, T., 1
Rich, M.W., 95
rise of managed care, 49–63
    Clinton plan, 62–63
    diversification, 55–57
    health maintenance organiza-
    tions, 51–55
    from minority to majority,
    60–61

new products, 57–59
opposition to, 50–51
trends, 61–62
risk adjustments, 157–58, 173, 174
in purchasing coalitions, 184
quality improvement, 198–199
Rodwin, M.A., 177

Salkever, D., 31
satisfaction levels, 134–35
satisfaction surveys, 112
Schuster, M.A., 134
scientific advances, 22–23
Scripps, 152
Scrushy, Richard, 113
selective contracting, 69–72, 83
self-insurers, 23, 57–59
definition, 18n
and ERISA, 175–76
plans, 175
selling quality, 155–58
Shadid, Michael, 49
shadow pricing, 55
shared decision-making, 92
Shaw, George Bernard, 6
shortcomings, 12–14
Shute, N., 123
Singer, S.J., 120
Siren, P.B., 88
Sloan, F.A., 31
Smith, Adam, 19
smoking cessation, 132, **133**, 191
socialism, 50
solo practitioners, 4, 37–38
specialists, 77–78, 139
growth of, 23
referrals to, 37, 123, **124**
surplus, 27–28, 28n
See also physicians
specialty benefit carve-outs, 97–98
specialty care, 77–78
spending, 1–4, **2**
spending per capita, 40–41

staff HMOs, 67–68, **67**. *See also*
HMOs; MCOs; traditional group
practice HMOs
standardization, 192
Stanford Medical Center University,
177
Starr, P., 25, 30, 49, 50
state cost controls, 31
state governments role, 176–77
state legislation, 104–5. *See also*
anti-managed care legislation
"State of Managed Care Quality,
The," (NCQA), 132–33
"State of Quality in Managed Care",
123
substance abuse services, 97
Sullivan, C.B., 1
supply and demand, 23–24, 139
surveys, 140
choice vs. costs, 147–48
medical profession, 38
symptomatic prostatic enlargement, 92

Take Care, 177–78, 201
tax deductions, 187–88
tax policy, 20–21, 187–88
teamwork, 87, 99
technological imperative, 23
Texas Board of Health, 163
Texas Heart Institute, 70
theory vs. practice, 12–14
tonsillectomies, 40
tools of managed care, case study,
82–85
track record, 119–136
blame the system, 121–23
consumer satisfaction, 134–35
costs, 120–21
fears, 123–26
marketplace, 126–28
quality, 129–34
value, 128–29
See also performance reports
trade-offs, 14–15, 23–25, 188–89

traditional group practice HMOs, 87, 99. *See also* HMOs; MCOs; staff model HMOs
traditional insurance, 106–7, 129–32
  and coalitions, 185
  failures of, 16–34
  flaws, 1–8
  payment system, 78–79
  See also fee-for-service; conventional health insurance
traditional medicine, 50–51
  cottage industry, 37–39, 42, 46
  education, 45–46
  flaws, 1–8
  and medical information, 42–43
  medical mistakes, 43–45
  physician accountability, 38–39
  practice variations, 39–42
  professionalism, 36–37, 41, 46–48
  quality, 35–48
  See also fee-for-service; traditional insurance
transurethral prostatectomy, 92
twenty-four-hour-stays, 168

UCLA (University of California, Los Angeles), 134
Ullman, 135
UM (utilization management). *See* utilization management
underutilization, 83–84
uninsured, 1
United HealthCare, 113

University of California Los Angeles (UCLA), 134
unnecessary procedures/services, 6–8, 73
U.S. Healthcare, 113, 143
"U.S. News and World Report," 147
utilization management (UM), 73–76
  capitation, 79–82
  gatekeepers, 76–78
  physician autonomy, 117
  prepayment, 78–82

value, 24–25, 128–29, 139–40
value-based choices, 186–87, **187**
value-based purchasing, 137–39
victory, pyrrhic, 31–32
voluntary efforts, 32

wage-price freeze, 30
wages, 1, 17–18
Wall Street analysts, 154–55
"Wall Street Journal," 119, 194
Ware, J.E., 131–32
"Washington Post," 119, 123
watchful waiting, 92
Wennberg, John, 40–41
Winslow, R., 195
Wisconsin statutes, 163

Zall, R.J., 163, 168
Zelman, Walter A., 19, 57